LOGICAL
NURSING
MATHEMATICS

Bruce Wilson, R.N., M.S.N.

Pan American University
Edinburg, Texas

 Delmar Publishers Inc.®

NOTICE TO THE READER

Delmar Staff
Administrative Editor: Leslie Boyer
Managing Editor: Barbara Christie
Production Editor: Ruth East
Design Coordinator: Susan Mathews

For information, address Delmar Publishers Inc.
2 Computer Drive West, Box 15-015
Albany, New York 12212

Printed in the United States of America
Published simultaneously in Canada
by Nelson Canada,
a division of International Thomson Limited

10 9 8 7 6 5 4 3 2 1

Library of Congress Cataloging in Publication Data

Wilson, Bruce, 1946-
  Logical nursing mathematics.

  Includes index.
  1. Nursing—Mathematics. 2. Pharmaceutical
arithmetic. 3. Medical logic. I. Title. [DNLM:
1. Mathematics—nurses' instruction. QA 107 W746L]
RT68.W55   1987   513'.024613   87-6824
ISBN 0-8273-2934-2 (soft)
ISBN 0-8273-2935-0 (instructor's guide)
ISBN 0-8273-2936-9 (diskette)

Contents

Preface

Nursing mathematics instruction can provide the opportunity for nursing students to learn logical and orderly thought processes. Most of nursing education has changed to teaching concepts instead of rote formulas. Likewise, *Logical Nursing Mathematics* teaches dosage calculations using the nursing process, and it teaches concepts instead of formula memorization and application. Nurses should think and not just follow formulas. *Logical Nursing Mathematics* teaches them to be logical and orderly thinkers, *especially* in mathematics, not *except* in mathematics.

The nursing process steps of assessment and analysis, planning, implementation, and evaluation are used in this book to guide the student to the correct answer. Because drug computation presents a wide variety of opportunities for logical problem solving, it also presents an ideal method for teaching and/or reinforcing the nursing process.

A reality faced by most programs is the necessity of reviewing basic arithmetic before being able to teach dosage calculations. Therefore, *Logical Nursing Mathematics* begins with a strong review of basic arithmetic principles. In Section I, the student learns the principles of the mathematical operation, not the terminology. For example, the phrase "dividend (number being divided)" is used instead of requiring the student to memorize the term "dividend."

In the second section, the student is taught that the first step in finding an answer is to identify the question. This is the assessment and analysis step of the nursing process. To promote this activity, problems presented in this book are purposely presented in several different formats. The student is required to identify the question within each problem, not just perform the calculations.

In the planning stage, the student must identify the information needed to solve the problem. This information may be given within the statement of the problem (i.e., one tablet contains 60 milligrams) or may be a standard conversion factor (i.e., 1000 mg = 1 g). The student also learns to disregard extraneous information.

The implementation stage, in which the student performs the mathematical calculations, is the only step most other nursing calculation books teach. By establishing the implementation stage as a separate step, this text distinguishes a student's arithmetic error from a problem-solving error and allows specific guidance to be provided.

Nursing mathematics is an excellent place to teach the importance of the evaluation stage of the nursing process. Even the best student sometimes makes an error. Students can learn, based upon their own actions, the ease with which mistakes are made and how evaluation can identify the error prior to a patient's being harmed.

Sections III and IV expand upon the logical thought processes. The student builds upon previously learned concepts and applies these concepts and processes to new situations.

The last unit of the book covers computers and calculators. In the real world, people use calculators to calculate more often than they use pencil and paper. This section helps the student identify and avoid common errors.

Logical Nursing Mathematics was developed after first identifying and questioning those nurses who perform medication calculations rapidly and accurately. These nurses typically do not use formulas, but instead follow a problem-solving process that provides faster, easier solutions. The author then began teaching the process to other nurses in both structured and unstructured settings. Numerous conversations with math teachers in non-nursing settings were part of the development process. Finally, the concepts were tested in the classroom and shared with other nursing educators. It is to all these individuals and to nursing students, who represent the future of nursing, that this book is dedicated.

Pretest Questions

The following questions provide the student with sample questions covering the content of each section. These questions may be used as an aid prior to studying the lessons or as a review before taking a section exam. The answers to the questions are located at the end of this book.

SECTION I

Work Space

(1) $\frac{1}{5} \times \frac{3}{8} = ?$

(2) $\frac{8}{15} \times \frac{4}{7} = ?$

(3) $\frac{3}{10} \times \frac{4}{7} \times \frac{2}{3} = ?$

(4) $\frac{1}{4} \div \frac{3}{8} = ?$

(5) $\dfrac{\frac{8}{15}}{\frac{4}{30}} = ?$

(6) $\dfrac{\frac{7}{32}}{5} = ?$

(7) $\frac{5}{8} + \frac{1}{8} = ?$

(8) $\frac{3}{12} + \frac{1}{6} = ?$

(9) $\frac{3}{10} + \frac{5}{7} + \frac{2}{3} = ?$

(10) $\frac{4}{5} - \frac{3}{8} = ?$

(11) $\frac{25}{31} - \frac{4}{9} = ?$

(12) $\frac{9}{10} - \frac{1}{8} - \frac{1}{3} = ?$

(13) $4 + \frac{7}{9} + \frac{8}{11} = ?$

(14) $52.65 + 32.58 = ?$

Work Space

(15) $4.036 + 1.2578 = ?$

(16) $3.2 - 1.5 = ?$

(17) $45.3 - 3.0578 = ?$

(18) $5.86 \times 3.2 = ?$

(19) $42 \times 3.657 = ?$

(20) $96 \div 19.2 = ?$

(21) $152.52 \div 24.6 = ?$

(22) Change $\dfrac{7}{8}$ into a decimal fraction.

(23) Change 125% into a regular fraction.

(24) Change $\dfrac{3}{5}$ into a percentage.

(25) $\dfrac{?}{40} = \dfrac{4}{32}$ $? =$ _____

(26) $\dfrac{57}{3} = \dfrac{76}{?}$ $? =$ _____

(27) If you can buy four cans of dog food for two dollars, how much would one can cost?

Work Space

(28) If you got 86% of the questions correct on a 50 question test, how many questions did you miss?

(29) If a baby drinks three ounces of milk every four hours, how many ounces will the baby drink each twenty-four hours?

(30) A runner completed a twenty-four mile marathon in 150 minutes. How many minutes did it take to run the average mile?

SECTION II

(1) You need to give Valium (Diazepam) 2.5 mg. You have tablets marked Valium 5 mg. How many tablets should you give?

(2) The physician's order reads, "Indocin 50 mg p.o. b.i.d." How many 25 mg capsules should you give in one dose?

(3) Mrs. A. is to receive Robaxin (Methocarbamol) 1 gram by mouth. 500 mg tablets are available. How many should you give?

(4) Mr. B. has an order for Cumadin 7.5 mg p.o. The tablets marked 5 mg/tab. How many tablets should you give?

(5) You have 250 mg Tetracycline capsules on the nursing unit. A physician has ordered 0.5 grams of Tetracycline p.o. for Miss C. How many capsules should be given?

(6) A patient is to receive Riopan (Magaldrate) 810 mg p.o. stat. The bottle reads, "Each 5 ml suspension contains: Magaldrate 540 mg." How many ml should be administered?

Work Space

(7) The physician has ordered Kantrex (Kanamycin Sulfate) 26.2 mg IM for John E. The Kantrex vial is labeled 75 mg per 2 ml. How many ml should you administer?

(8) Mr. G. should receive Erythromycin 800 mg p.o. q.6h. The bottle states 400 mg/5 cc. How many ml should he be given?

(9) Jane H. is to get 200 mg of Zarontin (Ethosuximide) by mouth q.d. How many ml should she receive when the medication is labeled 250 mg/5 ml?

(10) How many ml of Nafcillin (Nafcil) should Juan I. receive if the physician ordered 400 mg IM and the vial states, "Nafcil 500 mg add 1.8 ml sterile water for injection for 2.0 ml resulting solution?

(11) Baby J. is to receive Lanoxin (Digoxin) 25 mcg p.o. q.d. The bottle states, 0.05 mg/ml. How many ml should this child be given?

(12) The penicillin vial states, "Add 19.6 ml of diluent to provide 50,000 U/ml; add 9.6 ml of diluent to provide 100,000 U/ml; add 4.6 ml of diluent to provide 200,000 U/ml; add 3.6 ml of diluent to provide 250,000 U/ml; add 1.6 ml of diluent to provide 500,000 U/ml." 19.6 ml diluent has been added. How many ml are required for a 40,000 U dose?

(13) The penicillin vial states, "Add 19.6 ml of diluent to provide 50,000 U/ml; add 9.6 ml of diluent to provide 100,000 U/ml; add 4.6 ml of diluent to provide 200,000 U/ml; add 3.6 ml of diluent to provide 250,000 U/ml; add 1.6 ml of diluent to provide 500,000 U/ml." 4.6 ml diluent has been added. How many ml are required for a 300,000 U dose?

(14) The order reads, "Give ACTH 30 U IM stat." The vial states 1 unit = 1 mg, 40 units per milliliter. How many ml should be given?

Work Space

SECTION III

(1) Ms. K. is to receive Codeine gr ss p.o. You have 15 mg tablets in the narcotic box. How many tablets should you give?

(2) Mr. L. has Atropine 0.7 mg SC stat ordered. The Atropine vial is labeled gr 1/60 per ml. How many ml should you administer?

(3) Baby M. is to receive Acetaminophen gr i p.o. The bottle states, "80 mg acetaminophen per $\frac{1}{2}$ teaspoon." How many ml should you give to Baby M.?

(4) Jimmy N. was told his incision was 15 cm long. He wants to know how many inches this is equal to. How many inches should you tell him?

(5) Mrs. O. drank eight ounces of water. How many cc of intake should you record on her I & O record?

(6) Mr. P. has been told his baby weighs 2.5 kg. He wants to know the weight in pounds and ounces. What should you tell him?

(7) You are to give 250 cc D5W IV to Baby Q. over a 12 hr. period. The infusion set provides 60 drops per ml. How many drops should fall each minute?

(8) The physician's order reads, "Ringers Lactate 100 ml/hr. IV." How many drops should fall each minute if the solution administration set gives 20 gtt/ml?

(9) The patient is to receive three liters IV of fluid each day. How many ml should be given each hour?

(10) It is now 10 A.M. One liter of IV fluid was started two hours ago. What time will it run out if it runs at a rate of 200 cc per hour?

Work Space

(11) Jane R. is to receive 300 cc packed cells IV in two hours. The administration set states, "10 drops = 1 ml." How many drops should fall each minute?

(12) Mrs. S. is to receive Pitocin (Oxytocin) at a rate of 4 micro units per minute IV. A 1000 cc bag of 0.9% NaCl with 10 units of Pitocin added is hanging. The administration set provides 60 gtt/ml. How many drops should fall each minute?

(13) Mr. T.'s IV contains 20,000 U Heparin in 1000 ml isotonic sodium chloride solution for infusion. His orders state the heparin should be given at a rate of 30,000 U per day. The IV set provides 20 gtt/ml. How many drops should fall each minute?

(14) Ms. U. is to receive 250 mg of Aminophylline in one hour. The IV solution is labeled "Aminophylline 250 mg in 100 cc D5W." The administration set states, "15 gtt = 1 ml." How many drops should fall each minute?

(15) A patient is to receive Tridil (Nitroglycerine) at a rate of 80 mcg/min. The solution set provides 60 gtt/ml, and the IV Bottle is labeled 50 mg of Tridil in 500 ml D5W. How many drops should fall each minute?

SECTION IV

(1) A child is to receive Amikin (Amikacin Sulfate) 5 mg/kg IM Q8H. The child weighs 25 kg. How many milligrams should be given?

(2) A child is to receive Antiminth (Pyrantel Pamoate) 10 mg per kg p.o. The child weighs 33 pounds. How many milligrams should be given?

(3) Julie V. weighs 15 kg, and she is to receive Reserpine 0.01 mg/kg/dose p.o. b.i.d. The bottle is labeled, "Reserpine Elixir 0.2 mg/4 ml." How many ml should be administered?

Work Space

(4) Jacob W. weighs 110 pounds and is to receive Amikin (Amikacin Sulfate) 7.5 mg/kg IM q.12h. The Amikin label states, "1.0 gm per 4 ml." How many ml should be given?

(5) Janice X. is to receive Ampicillin 250 mg IV over a 20 minute period. Her IV is running at 30 cc per hour, and the administration set gives 60 gtt/ml. How many cc should she receive with the Ampicillin?

(6) Jack Y. has an order for Demerol (Meperidine HCl) 50 mg IM q.4h. p.r.n. Your drug reference states the dosage range is 0.5-0.8 mg/kg q. 3-4 hr. Is this amount safe if Jack weighs only 88 pounds?

(7) Jill Z. is to receive Isoniazid 1 tab. q.d. Jill weighs 50 pounds, and the tablets are labeled, "Isoniazid 300 mg." Your drug reference states the dosage range is 10 to 30 mg per kg. Can the ordered amount endanger Jill?

(8) The physician orders 50 mg Nipride (Sodium Nitroprusside) to be mixed in 500 ml D5W and given at a rate of 60 drops per minute with an administration set giving 20 gtt/ml. The patient weighs 176 pounds, and your drug reference states a rate of 10 mcg/kg/min. should not be exceeded. Should the physician's order be questioned?

(9) A woman in labor is receiving Magnesium Sulfate 4 gm in 250 cc D5W at a rate of 30 drops per minute. The administration set provides 20 drops/ml. The OB policies state a rate over 3 gm/hr should not be administered. Is this amount in excess of 3 gm/hr?

(10) A child has a body surface area of 0.75 m^2, and is to receive Cleocin (Clindamycin Phosphate) IM at a rate of 400 mg/m^2/day divided into four doses. How many milligrams will be in each dose?

(11) Julio A. weighs 30 kg and is to receive Lincocin (Lincomycin) IM q.12h at a rate of 15 mg/kg/day. How many ml will Julio receive in each dose if Lincocin comes in 300 mg/2 cc?

Work Space

(12) How many °F is 41°C?

(13) How many °F is 32°C?

(14) How many °C is 104°F?

(15) How many °C is 86°F?

(16) How many grams of dextrose are in 500 cc of 5% dextrose in water?

(17) How many ml of Similac 20 cal/1 oz should be used to make 90 ml of a 10 cal/1 oz solution?

Section **I**
MATHEMATICS REVIEW

Unit One
Speaking in Measurements

Let's imagine for a moment that you are trying to get a job in a hospital that refused to use measurements.

> Personnel Director: "You've got the job."
> You: "When do I start?"
> Personnel Director: "Sometime."
> You: "What will I do?"
> Personnel Director: "Something."
> You: "Where will I work?"
> Personnel Director: "Somewhere."
> You: "What will I be paid?"
> Personnel Director: "Some money."

There are times when "some" isn't an adequate answer. Measurement is a part of life. From the simplest to the most complex living organisms, measurement is a way of evaluating and responding to their surroundings.

Measurement consists of two areas: (1) the types of units used in measuring, and (2) the number of those units. A dime can be described as a dime or as one tenth of a dollar or as ten cents. In each case, the amount of money remains the same but both the *type* of unit and the *number* of those units has changed. In health care, you will frequently have to change both the number of units being used and the type of those units in order to provide good patient care.

EQUATIONS

An equation describes a balance on each side of an equals (=) sign. The equation may be written in words (as in one dime equals ten cents) or in symbols (as in $0.10 = 10¢) or with a symbol representing an unknown quantity (as in $0.10 = ? ¢). Frequently, the Greek letter chi (χ) is used to represent an unknown quantity. In these materials, the question mark symbol (?) will be used. In all equations, the user must remember to keep the equation in balance.

The user must also remember that the equation may deal with measurements of only one aspect of the items being measured. For example, if you've ever faced a vending machine without the proper change, you know that ten pennies do not equal one dime. The machine evaluates the size and weight of the inserted coins, not their value. The user of the equation must keep in mind what is being measured and what the measurements mean.

It is possible to use an equation to equate two very different aspects of one item. When we say a car is traveling 50 miles per hour, an equation is being used that equates distance and time. The item the equation is based upon is the rate of speed for that car. The word "per" is Latin and means *for each, for every,* or *equals.* The symbolic form of this equation is "50 miles = 1 hour." For that car traveling at that rate of speed, every 50 miles will take 1 hour of travel time, and for every hour spent traveling, a distance of fifty miles will be covered.

The yield symbol ($\rightarrow$) may be used in place of the equals sign (=). This commonly occurs in computations where the use of equal signs would be confusing. For example, 50 miles/1 hour $\rightarrow$ speed of car.

When working with equations always remember (1) what is being equated and (2) to keep the equation in balance.

ADDITION AND SUBTRACTION

Addition is the process of combining things. Whoever said you can't mix apples and oranges didn't try putting them in the same box. You *can* add five apples and five oranges. However, the total will not be in units of "apples" or of "oranges," but must be expressed in terms of "pieces of fruit." Subtraction is the process of taking something away. In mathematics, you can take something away even if it isn't there to begin with. This process is like borrowing money. You go into debt for the amount you need minus the amount you have.

MULTIPLICATION

Multiplication is merely fast addition of a number. The number is added to itself a specific number of times. Five times three is the same thing as $5 + 5 + 5$. In fact, computers don't do multiplication, they only do addition at a very fast rate. Multiplying any number by one doesn't change the quantity; five times one is five.

Several words and symbols are used to indicate multiplication:

Word or Symbol	**Example**
of	four *of* those dimes is $0.40
times	four *times* a dime is $0.40
×	$4 \times 10¢ = \$0.40$
*	$4 * 10¢ = \$0.40$
( )( )	$(4)(10¢) = \$0.40$

DIVISION

Division is the process of separating one amount into an *equal* number of parts. For example, if we divide 6 dollars equally among 2 children, each child would get 3 dollars.

Just as any amount can be multiplied by one without changing the amount, any amount can be divided by one without changing the amount.

Several words and symbols are used to indicate division:

Word or Symbol	Example
for	4 apples for 2 children
/	4 apples/2 children
———	$\dfrac{4 \text{ apples}}{2 \text{ children}}$
÷	4 apples ÷ 2 children
⌐	2 children $\overline{)4 \text{ apples}}$

Unit Two
Fractions

A fraction is a measurement that indicates division is occurring. The top number (the numerator) represents the initial number of parts or items. The bottom number (the denominator) represents the number that is doing the dividing. For example, $\frac{1}{2}$ dollar is equal to 1 of the parts when 1 dollar is divided into 2 parts, and $\frac{3}{4}$ dollar is equal to 3 of the parts when 1 dollar is divided into 4 parts. The unit of measurement (in this example a dollar) can be written after the fraction, but it refers to only the top number (numerator).

MULTIPLYING FRACTIONS

First, remember that multiplication is taking a number and adding it to itself a specific number of times. In order to multiply fractions you must (1) multiply the top numbers (numerators) and that result becomes the new top number (numerator), then (2) multiply the bottom numbers (denominators) and that result becomes the new bottom number (denominator). For example:

$$\frac{1}{2} \text{ dollar} \times \frac{1}{2} = \frac{1 \text{ dollar} \times 1}{2 \times 2} = \frac{1}{4} \text{ dollar}$$

In this case, we are taking one half ($\frac{1}{2}$) of one half ($\frac{1}{2}$) dollar. The answer is *less* than the original amount because the original amount ($\frac{1}{2}$ dollar) was added *less* than one full time. Other examples are:

$$\frac{5}{6} \text{ apples} \times \frac{5}{8} = \frac{5 \text{ apples} \times 5}{6 \times 8} = \frac{25}{48} \text{ apples}$$

and

$$\frac{7}{6} \times \frac{3}{2} = \frac{7 \times 3}{6 \times 2} = \frac{21}{12}$$

☛ **HINTS AND REMINDERS:** In the last example, the resulting fraction is greater than the initial fractions because the initial fractions were greater than 1.

Exercise 1

The answers to the following problems are located at the end of this unit. Complete one set of problems, then check your answers. If you are unable to complete the problems *or* if you complete all the sets but don't score 100% on any set, SEE THE INSTRUCTOR. You *do not* need to complete all the sets *if* you can complete a set with 100% correct and understand the principles.

Set 1

(a) $\frac{3}{4} \times \frac{6}{7} = ?$

(b) $\frac{9}{16} \times \frac{7}{8} = ?$

(c) $\frac{5}{11} \times \frac{3}{4} = ?$

(d) $\frac{12}{10} \times \frac{8}{3} = ?$

(e) $\frac{32}{81} \times \frac{17}{23} = ?$

Set 2

(a) $\frac{2}{7} \times \frac{1}{4} = ?$

(b) $\frac{1}{44} \times \frac{9}{6} = ?$

(c) $\frac{3}{57} \times \frac{3}{5} = ?$

(d) $\frac{28}{57} \times \frac{6}{7} = ?$

(e) $\frac{98}{16} \times \frac{19}{67} = ?$

Set 3

(a) $\frac{7}{4} \times \frac{6}{9} = ?$

(b) $\frac{2}{81} \times \frac{5}{7} = ?$

(c) $\frac{2}{65} \times \frac{8}{9} = ?$

(d) $\frac{14}{59} \times \frac{7}{2} = ?$

(e) $\frac{44}{37} \times \frac{37}{16} = ?$

Work Space

DIVIDING FRACTIONS

☛ **HINTS AND REMINDERS:** A fraction is an expression of division.

Division of a fraction is the process of dividing something that is already being divided. This process is accomplished by (1) inverting the lower fraction and then (2) multiplying the resulting fractions. For example:

$$\frac{\frac{1}{2} \text{ dollar}}{\frac{1}{2}} = \frac{1 \text{ dollar}}{2} \times \frac{2}{1} = \frac{2}{2} \text{ dollar}$$

or

$$\frac{1}{2} \text{ dollar} \div \frac{1}{2} = \frac{1 \text{ dollar}}{2} \times \frac{2}{1} = \frac{2}{2} \text{ dollar}$$

If the number divided into the fraction is not a fraction (i.e., it is a whole number), the number can be turned into a fraction by dividing it by 1.

Any number can be divided by 1 or multiplied by 1 without changing the amount it represents. For example:

$$5 \div 1 = 5$$

or

$$\frac{3}{5} \div 5 = \frac{3}{5} \times \frac{1}{5} = \frac{3}{25}$$

or

$$\frac{\frac{4}{10}}{2} \rightarrow \frac{\frac{4}{10}}{\frac{2}{1}} \rightarrow \frac{4}{10} \times \frac{1}{2} = \frac{4}{20}$$

☛ **HINTS AND REMINDERS:** In the above equation, the yield symbol ($\rightarrow$) is used in place of an equal sign.

Exercise 2

The answers to the following problems are located at the end of this unit. Complete one set of problems, then check your answers. If you are unable to complete the problems *or* if you complete all the sets but don't score 100% on any set, SEE THE INSTRUCTOR. You *do not* need to complete all the sets *if* you can complete a set with 100% correct and understand the principles.

Set 1

(a) $\frac{3}{4} \div \frac{6}{7} = ?$

(b) $\frac{9}{16} \div \frac{7}{8} = ?$

(c) $\frac{5}{11} \div \frac{3}{4} = ?$

(d) $\frac{12}{10} \div \frac{8}{3} = ?$

(e) $\frac{32}{81} \div \frac{17}{23} = ?$

(f) $\frac{45}{81} \div 2 = ?$

Set 2

(a) $\frac{2}{7} \div \frac{1}{4} = ?$

(b) $\frac{1}{44} \div \frac{9}{6} = ?$

(c) $\frac{3}{57} \div \frac{3}{5} = ?$

(d) $\frac{28}{57} \div \frac{6}{7} = ?$

(e) $\frac{98}{16} \div \frac{19}{67} = ?$

(f) $\frac{55}{23} \div 3 = ?$

Set 3

(a) $\frac{7}{4} \div \frac{6}{9} = ?$

(b) $\frac{2}{81} \div \frac{5}{7} = ?$

(c) $\frac{2}{65} \div \frac{8}{9} = ?$

(d) $\frac{14}{59} \div \frac{7}{2} = ?$

(e) $\frac{44}{37} \div \frac{37}{16} = ?$

(f) $\frac{58}{12} \div 4 = ?$

Work Space

ADDING AND SUBTRACTING FRACTIONS

A key point to remember in adding or subtracting fractions is that you *only* add or subtract the top numbers (numerators) if the bottom numbers (denominators) are the same. For example:

$$\frac{1}{2} \text{ dollar } + \frac{1}{2} \text{ dollar } = \frac{2}{2} \text{ dollar}$$

and

$$\frac{1}{2} \text{ dollar } - \frac{1}{2} \text{ dollar } = \frac{0}{2} \text{ dollar}$$

☞ **HINTS AND REMINDERS:** Because fractions are a division process, 2 dollars divided into 2 parts is equal to 1 dollar, and 0 dollars divided into 2 parts is still 0 dollars.

If the bottom numbers (denominators) are not the same, the fractions cannot be added or subtracted until the bottom numbers (denominators) become the same. This is called having a *common denominator*. For example, we want to add $\frac{1}{2}$ circle and $\frac{1}{4}$ circle. The equation would be written "$\frac{1}{2}$ circle $+ \frac{1}{4}$ circle $= ?$ circle." Visually, the equation looks like:

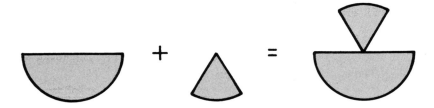

Any number divided by itself equals 1 (for example, $\frac{2}{2} = 1$, $\frac{3}{3} = 1$, $\frac{4}{4} = 1$, etc.) and any number can be multiplied by 1 without changing the quantity it represents (for example, $2 \times 1 = 2$, $3 \times 1 = 3$, $4 \times 1 = 4$, etc.). Therefore, we can multiply a fraction by a fraction with the same top number (numerator) and the same bottom number (denominator) without changing the quantity the initial fraction represents. If we use the example $\frac{1}{2}$ circle $+ \frac{1}{4}$ circle $= ?$ circle, we first multiply $\frac{1}{2}$ circle $\times$ $\frac{2}{2} = \frac{2}{4}$ circle. Then we have a common denominator and can add the fractions.

$$\frac{2}{4} \text{ circle} + \frac{1}{4} \text{ circle} = \frac{3}{4} \text{ circle}$$

Visually, the equation looks like:

One way of finding a common denominator is to use the bottom number (denominator) of the other numbers as the top number (numerator) and the top number (numerator) of the fraction you are multiplying with. Remember, once the common denominator is identified, *only* the top numbers (numerators) are added or subtracted. For example:

$$\frac{1}{2} + \frac{1}{4} \;\rightarrow\; \frac{1 \times 4}{2 \times 4} + \frac{1 \times 2}{4 \times 2} \;\rightarrow\; \frac{4}{8} + \frac{2}{8} = \frac{6}{8}$$

When there are more than two fractions to be added (or subtracted), each of the bottom numbers (denominators) can be used to determine a common bottom number (denominator). For example:

$$
\begin{array}{rcll}
& \dfrac{1}{3} & \dfrac{1 \times 7 \times 8}{3 \times 7 \times 8} & \dfrac{56}{168} \\[3ex]
+ & \dfrac{1}{7} \;\rightarrow\; & \dfrac{1 \times 3 \times 8}{7 \times 3 \times 8} \;\rightarrow\; & \dfrac{24}{168} \\[3ex]
+ & \dfrac{5}{8} & \dfrac{5 \times 3 \times 8}{8 \times 3 \times 7} & \dfrac{105}{168} \\
\hline
& & & \dfrac{182}{168}
\end{array}
$$

Exercise 3

The answers to the following problems are located at the end of this unit. Complete one set of problems, then check your answers. If you are unable to complete the problems *or* if you complete all the sets but don't score 100% on any set, SEE THE INSTRUCTOR. You *do not* need to complete all the sets *if* you can complete a set with 100% correct and understand the principles.

Set 1	Set 2	**Work Space**
(a) $\frac{3}{4} + \frac{6}{7} = ?$	(a) $\frac{2}{7} + \frac{1}{4} = ?$	
(b) $\frac{9}{16} + \frac{7}{8} = ?$	(b) $\frac{1}{44} + \frac{9}{6} = ?$	
(c) $\frac{5}{11} + \frac{3}{4} = ?$	(c) $\frac{3}{57} + \frac{3}{5} = ?$	
(d) $\frac{12}{10} + \frac{8}{3} = ?$	(d) $\frac{28}{57} + \frac{6}{7} = ?$	
(e) $\frac{32}{81} + \frac{17}{23} + \frac{3}{4} = ?$	(e) $\frac{98}{16} + \frac{19}{67} + \frac{4}{7} = ?$	
(f) $\frac{3}{4} - \frac{1}{7} = ?$	(f) $\frac{3}{7} - \frac{1}{4} = ?$	
(g) $\frac{9}{16} - \frac{3}{8} = ?$	(g) $\frac{21}{44} - \frac{1}{6} = ?$	
(h) $\frac{15}{11} - \frac{3}{4} = ?$	(h) $\frac{53}{57} - \frac{3}{5} = ?$	
(i) $\frac{12}{10} - \frac{2}{3} = ?$	(i) $\frac{28}{57} - \frac{1}{7} = ?$	
(j) $\frac{32}{81} - \frac{7}{23} = ?$	(j) $\frac{98}{16} - \frac{19}{67} = ?$	

Set 3   **Work Space**

(a) $\frac{7}{4} + \frac{6}{9} = ?$

(b) $\frac{2}{81} + \frac{5}{7} = ?$

(c) $\frac{2}{65} + \frac{8}{9} = ?$

(d) $\frac{14}{59} + \frac{7}{2} = ?$

(e) $\frac{44}{37} + \frac{37}{16} + \frac{5}{3} = ?$

(f) $\frac{7}{4} - \frac{6}{9} = ?$

(g) $\frac{22}{81} - \frac{1}{7} = ?$

(h) $\frac{62}{65} - \frac{8}{9} = ?$

(i) $\frac{44}{59} - \frac{1}{2} = ?$

(j) $\frac{44}{37} - \frac{15}{16} = ?$

REDUCING FRACTIONS

In the previous section, we expanded the fractions to get a common denominator. After the calculations (addition, subtraction, multiplication, and/or division) have been completed, it is necessary to reduce the answer to the simplest form. Fractions are reduced in order to prevent confusion and unnecessary calculations. It is much easier to work with $\frac{1}{3}$ of something than to work with $\frac{56}{168}$ ths of something even though both fractions indicate the same quantity.

The method for reducing fractions is just the opposite of the method used to expand fractions. Instead of multiplying the top number (numerator) and the bottom number (denominator) by the same amount, we divide the top number (numerator) and the bottom number (denominator) by the same amount.

Expansion   **Reduction**

$$\frac{1 \times 4}{3 \times 4} = \frac{4}{12} \qquad \frac{4 \div 4}{12 \div 4} = \frac{1}{3}$$

A simple way of determining if a fraction can be reduced is to attempt to divide both numbers by 2, then 3, then 5, then 7, then 11, then 13, then 17 to see if any of these numbers will divide evenly (leaving no remainder) into the top number (numerator) *and* the bottom number (denominator).

☞ **HINTS AND REMINDERS:** If both the top number (numerator) and the bottom number (denominator) end in a 0, the number is divisible by 10; if the top number (numerator) and the bottom number (denominator) end in either a 5 or a 0, the number is divisible by 5.

The process is repeated until no number is found that will divide evenly into the top number (numerator) and the bottom number (denominator). For example:

$$\frac{56 \div 2}{168 \div 2} = \frac{28 \div 2}{84 \div 2} = \frac{14 \div 2}{42 \div 2} = \frac{7 \div 7}{21 \div 7} = \frac{1}{3}$$

One easy way of writing this is to first write the fraction, then after finding a number that will evenly divide into the top number (numerator) and the bottom number (denominator), draw a line through the initial numbers and write the new top number (numerator) and bottom number (denominator). For example:

$$\begin{array}{c} 1 \\ \cancel{7} \\ \cancel{14} \\ \cancel{28} \\ \cancel{56} \\ \overline{\cancel{168}} \\ \cancel{84} \\ \cancel{42} \\ \cancel{21} \\ 3 \end{array}$$

Exercise 4

Try reducing the following fractions. Complete one set of problems, then check your answers at the end of the unit. If you are unable to complete the problems *or* complete all the sets without being able to score 100% on any set, SEE THE INSTRUCTOR. You *do not* need to complete all the sets *if* you can complete a set with 100% correct and understand the principles.

Set 1

(a) $\frac{14}{21} = ?$

(b) $\frac{20}{75} = ?$

(c) $\frac{36}{60} = ?$

(d) $\frac{24}{72} = ?$

Set 2

(a) $\frac{33}{55} = ?$

(b) $\frac{18}{45} = ?$

(c) $\frac{12}{60} = ?$

(d) $\frac{26}{65} = ?$

Set 3

(a) $\frac{17}{68} = ?$

(b) $\frac{32}{64} = ?$

(c) $\frac{9}{27} = ?$

(d) $\frac{45}{66} = ?$

Work Space

MIXED NUMBERS

A mixed number is a combination of a whole number (i.e., 1, 2, 3, 4, etc.) and a fraction; for example, two and one fourth ($2\frac{1}{4}$). The word "and" indicates that an addition process is taking place. This mixed number could also be written as $2 + \frac{1}{4}$.

When it is necessary to convert a mixed number into a fraction, you simply follow the rules for adding fractions.

$$2 + \frac{1}{4} \rightarrow \frac{2}{1} + \frac{1}{4} \rightarrow \frac{2 \times 4}{1 \times 4} + \frac{1}{4} \rightarrow \frac{8}{4} + \frac{1}{4} = \frac{9}{4}$$

When a mixed number is converted into a fraction, it becomes an *improper fraction*. An improper fraction exists any time the top number (numerator) is larger than the bottom number (denominator). Improper numbers need to be reduced for the same reasons expanded numbers need to be reduced. To reduce an improper fraction, the top number (numerator) is divided by the bottom number (denominator) until no further whole numbers can be obtained. The remainder (amount left over) then becomes the new top number (numerator) and is placed over the original bottom number (denominator). For example:

$$\frac{7}{3} \rightarrow 3\overline{\smash{\big)}7}\begin{array}{c} 2\frac{1}{3} \\ \hline \end{array} \rightarrow 2\frac{1}{3}$$
$$\frac{6}{1}$$

and

$$\frac{65}{4} \rightarrow 4\overline{\smash{\big)}65}\begin{array}{c} 16\frac{1}{4} \\ \hline \end{array} \rightarrow 16\frac{1}{4}$$
$$\frac{4}{25}$$
$$\frac{24}{1}$$

In a previous example we found that

$$\frac{1}{3} + \frac{1}{7} + \frac{5}{8} = \frac{182}{168}$$

$\frac{182}{168}$ is an improper fraction and needs to be reduced.

$$\frac{182}{168} \rightarrow 168\overline{\smash{\big)}182}\begin{array}{c} 1\frac{14}{168} \\ \hline \end{array} = 1\frac{14}{168}$$
$$\frac{168}{14}$$

$1\frac{14}{168}$ needs to be reduced further since $\frac{14}{168}$ is an expanded fraction.

$$\frac{14 \text{ (divided by 2)}}{168 \text{ (divided by 2)}} \rightarrow \frac{7 \text{ (divided by 7)}}{84 \text{ (divided by 7)}} \rightarrow \frac{1}{12}$$

The simplest answer to $\frac{1}{3} + \frac{1}{7} + \frac{5}{8}$ is $1\frac{1}{12}$.

Exercise 5

Try reducing the following fractions to their simplest form. Complete one set of problems, then check your answers at the end of the unit. If you are unable to complete the problems *or* if you complete all the sets but don't score 100% on any set, SEE THE INSTRUCTOR. You *do not* need to complete all the sets *if* you can complete a set with 100% correct and understand the principles.

Set 1

(a) $\frac{54}{21} = ?$

(b) $\frac{90}{75} = ?$

(c) $\frac{86}{60} = ?$

(d) $\frac{24}{22} = ?$

Set 2

(a) $\frac{95}{55} = ?$

(b) $\frac{18}{13} = ?$

(c) $\frac{60}{12} = ?$

(d) $\frac{26}{5} = ?$

Set 3

(a) $\frac{68}{17} = ?$

(b) $\frac{62}{33} = ?$

(c) $\frac{99}{27} = ?$

(d) $\frac{45}{6} = ?$

Work Space

You don't need to wait until the answer is obtained in order to begin reducing fractions. Any time fractions are multiplied, compare all the top numbers (numerators) with all the bottom numbers (denominators) and reduce the numbers at that time. It will simplify both the process of multiplying the fractions and the process of reducing the answer. For example:

$$\frac{2}{5} \times \frac{15}{22} \rightarrow \frac{\overset{1}{\cancel{2}}}{\underset{1}{\cancel{5}}} \times \frac{\overset{3}{\cancel{15}}}{\underset{11}{\cancel{22}}} = \frac{3}{11}$$

For additional examples, lets look at problems a and b of Set 2 of Exercise 1:

$$(a)\quad \frac{2}{7} \times \frac{1}{4} \rightarrow \frac{\overset{1}{\cancel{2}}}{7} \times \frac{1}{\underset{2}{\cancel{4}}} = \frac{1}{14}$$

$$(b)\quad \frac{1}{44} \times \frac{9}{6} \rightarrow \frac{1}{44} \times \frac{\overset{3}{\cancel{9}}}{\underset{2}{\cancel{6}}} = \frac{3}{88}$$

By reducing fractions as early as possible, you avoid multiplying by a number and then dividing by the same number. This helps eliminate mistakes because (a) it eliminates an extra calculation and (b) you work with smaller numbers. For example, the following problem can be worked in two ways:

$$\frac{3}{5} \times \frac{15}{22} \times \frac{4}{9} \rightarrow \frac{\overset{2}{\cancel{6}}\overset{}{\cancel{18}}\cancel{180}}{\underset{11}{\cancel{990}\cancel{99}\cancel{33}}} \rightarrow \frac{2}{11}$$

or

$$\overset{1}{\underset{1}{\cancel{\frac{3}{5}}}} \times \overset{\overset{1}{\cancel{3}}}{\underset{11}{\cancel{\frac{15}{22}}}} \times \overset{2}{\underset{\underset{1}{\cancel{3}}}{\cancel{\frac{4}{9}}}} = \frac{2}{11}$$

You can practice reducing while multiplying on any of the sets in Exercise 1 or Exercise 2. Remember that in division you invert before you reduce.

Answers to Exercises
Exercise 1

Set 1

(a) $\frac{3}{4} \times \frac{6}{7} = \frac{18}{28}$

(b) $\frac{9}{16} \times \frac{7}{8} = \frac{63}{128}$

(c) $\frac{5}{11} \times \frac{3}{4} = \frac{15}{44}$

(d) $\frac{12}{10} \times \frac{8}{3} = \frac{96}{30}$

(e) $\frac{32}{81} \times \frac{17}{23} = \frac{544}{1863}$

Set 2

(a) $\frac{2}{7} \times \frac{1}{4} = \frac{2}{28}$

(b) $\frac{1}{44} \times \frac{9}{6} = \frac{9}{264}$

(c) $\frac{3}{57} \times \frac{3}{5} = \frac{9}{285}$

(d) $\frac{28}{57} \times \frac{6}{7} = \frac{168}{399}$

(e) $\frac{98}{16} \times \frac{19}{67} = \frac{1862}{1072}$

Set 3

(a) $\frac{7}{4} \times \frac{6}{9} = \frac{42}{36}$

(b) $\frac{2}{81} \times \frac{5}{7} = \frac{10}{567}$

(c) $\frac{2}{65} \times \frac{8}{9} = \frac{16}{585}$

(d) $\frac{14}{59} \times \frac{7}{2} = \frac{98}{118}$

(e) $\frac{44}{37} \times \frac{37}{16} = \frac{1628}{592}$

Exercise 2

Set 1

(a) $\dfrac{3}{4} \div \dfrac{6}{7} = \dfrac{3}{4} \times \dfrac{7}{6} = \dfrac{21}{24}$

(b) $\dfrac{9}{16} \div \dfrac{7}{8} = \dfrac{9}{16} \times \dfrac{8}{7} = \dfrac{72}{112}$

(c) $\dfrac{5}{11} \div \dfrac{3}{4} = \dfrac{5}{11} \times \dfrac{4}{3} = \dfrac{20}{33}$

(d) $\dfrac{12}{10} \div \dfrac{8}{3} = \dfrac{12}{10} \times \dfrac{3}{8} = \dfrac{36}{80}$

(e) $\dfrac{32}{81} \div \dfrac{17}{23} = \dfrac{32}{81} \times \dfrac{23}{17} = \dfrac{736}{1377}$

(f) $\dfrac{45}{81} \div 2 = \dfrac{45}{81} \times \dfrac{1}{2} = \dfrac{45}{162}$

Set 2

(a) $\dfrac{2}{7} \div \dfrac{1}{4} = \dfrac{8}{7}$

(b) $\dfrac{1}{44} \div \dfrac{9}{6} = \dfrac{6}{396}$

(c) $\dfrac{3}{57} \div \dfrac{3}{5} = \dfrac{15}{171}$

(d) $\dfrac{28}{57} \div \dfrac{6}{7} = \dfrac{196}{342}$

(e) $\dfrac{98}{16} \div \dfrac{19}{67} = \dfrac{6566}{304}$

(f) $\dfrac{55}{23} \div 3 = \dfrac{55}{69}$

Set 3

(a) $\dfrac{7}{4} \div \dfrac{6}{9} = \dfrac{63}{24}$

(b) $\dfrac{2}{81} \div \dfrac{5}{7} = \dfrac{14}{405}$

(c) $\dfrac{2}{65} \div \dfrac{8}{9} = \dfrac{18}{520}$

(d) $\dfrac{14}{59} \div \dfrac{7}{2} = \dfrac{28}{413}$

(e) $\dfrac{44}{37} \div \dfrac{37}{16} = \dfrac{704}{1369}$

(f) $\dfrac{58}{12} \div 4 = \dfrac{58}{48}$

Exercise 3

Set 1

(a) $\dfrac{3}{4} + \dfrac{6}{7} = \dfrac{3 \times 7}{4 \times 7} + \dfrac{6 \times 4}{7 \times 4} = \dfrac{21}{28} + \dfrac{24}{28} = \dfrac{45}{28}$

(b) $\dfrac{9}{16} + \dfrac{7}{8} = \dfrac{9 \times 8}{16 \times 8} + \dfrac{7 \times 16}{8 \times 16} = \dfrac{72}{128} + \dfrac{112}{128} = \dfrac{184}{128}$

(c) $\dfrac{5}{11} + \dfrac{3}{4} = \dfrac{5 \times 4}{11 \times 4} + \dfrac{3 \times 11}{4 \times 11} = \dfrac{20}{44} + \dfrac{33}{44} = \dfrac{53}{44}$

(d) $\dfrac{12}{10} + \dfrac{8}{3} = \dfrac{12 \times 3}{10 \times 3} + \dfrac{8 \times 10}{3 \times 10} = \dfrac{36}{30} + \dfrac{80}{30} = \dfrac{116}{30}$

(e) $\dfrac{32}{81} + \dfrac{17}{23} + \dfrac{3}{4} = \dfrac{32 \times 23 \times 4}{81 \times 23 \times 4} + \dfrac{17 \times 81 \times 4}{23 \times 81 \times 4} + \dfrac{3 \times 81 \times 23}{4 \times 81 \times 23} =$

$\dfrac{2944}{7452} + \dfrac{5508}{7452} + \dfrac{5589}{7452} = \dfrac{14041}{7452}$

(f) $\dfrac{3}{4} - \dfrac{1}{7} = \dfrac{3 \times 7}{4 \times 7} - \dfrac{1 \times 4}{7 \times 4} = \dfrac{21}{28} - \dfrac{4}{28} = \dfrac{17}{28}$

(g) $\dfrac{9}{16} - \dfrac{3}{8} = \dfrac{9 \times 8}{16 \times 8} - \dfrac{3 \times 16}{8 \times 16} = \dfrac{72}{128} - \dfrac{48}{128} = \dfrac{24}{128}$

(h) $\dfrac{15}{11} - \dfrac{3}{4} = \dfrac{15 \times 4}{11 \times 4} - \dfrac{3 \times 11}{4 \times 11} = \dfrac{60}{44} - \dfrac{33}{44} = \dfrac{27}{44}$

(i) $\dfrac{12}{10} - \dfrac{2}{3} = \dfrac{12 \times 3}{10 \times 3} - \dfrac{2 \times 10}{3 \times 10} = \dfrac{36}{30} - \dfrac{20}{30} = \dfrac{16}{30}$

(j) $\dfrac{32}{81} - \dfrac{7}{23} = \dfrac{32 \times 23}{81 \times 23} - \dfrac{7 \times 81}{23 \times 81} = \dfrac{736}{1863} - \dfrac{567}{1863} = \dfrac{169}{1863}$

Set 2

(a) $\dfrac{2}{7} + \dfrac{1}{4} = \dfrac{15}{28}$

(b) $\dfrac{1}{44} + \dfrac{9}{6} = \dfrac{402}{264}$

(c) $\dfrac{3}{57} + \dfrac{3}{5} = \dfrac{186}{285}$

(d) $\dfrac{28}{57} + \dfrac{6}{7} = \dfrac{538}{399}$

(e) $\dfrac{98}{16} + \dfrac{19}{67} + \dfrac{4}{7} = \dfrac{52378}{7504}$

(f) $\dfrac{3}{7} - \dfrac{1}{4} = \dfrac{5}{28}$

(g) $\dfrac{21}{44} - \dfrac{1}{6} = \dfrac{82}{264}$

(h) $\dfrac{53}{57} - \dfrac{3}{5} = \dfrac{94}{285}$

(i) $\dfrac{28}{57} - \dfrac{1}{7} = \dfrac{139}{399}$

(j) $\dfrac{98}{16} - \dfrac{19}{67} = \dfrac{6262}{1072}$

Set 3

(a) $\dfrac{7}{4} + \dfrac{6}{9} = \dfrac{87}{36}$

(b) $\dfrac{2}{81} + \dfrac{5}{7} = \dfrac{419}{567}$

(c) $\dfrac{2}{65} + \dfrac{8}{9} = \dfrac{538}{585}$

(d) $\dfrac{14}{59} + \dfrac{7}{2} = \dfrac{441}{118}$

(e) $\dfrac{44}{37} + \dfrac{37}{16} + \dfrac{5}{3} = \dfrac{9179}{1776}$

(f) $\dfrac{7}{4} - \dfrac{6}{9} = \dfrac{39}{36}$

(g) $\dfrac{22}{81} - \dfrac{1}{7} = \dfrac{73}{567}$

(h) $\dfrac{62}{65} - \dfrac{8}{9} = \dfrac{38}{585}$

(i) $\dfrac{44}{59} - \dfrac{1}{2} = \dfrac{29}{118}$

(j) $\dfrac{44}{37} - \dfrac{15}{16} = \dfrac{149}{592}$

Exercise 4

Set 1

(a) $\dfrac{14}{21} = \dfrac{2}{3}$

(b) $\dfrac{20}{75} = \dfrac{4}{15}$

(c) $\dfrac{36}{60} = \dfrac{3}{5}$

(d) $\dfrac{24}{72} = \dfrac{1}{3}$

Set 2

(a) $\dfrac{33}{55} = \dfrac{3}{5}$

(b) $\dfrac{18}{45} = \dfrac{2}{5}$

(c) $\dfrac{12}{60} = \dfrac{1}{5}$

(d) $\dfrac{26}{65} = \dfrac{2}{5}$

Set 3

(a) $\dfrac{17}{68} = \dfrac{1}{4}$

(b) $\dfrac{32}{64} = \dfrac{1}{2}$

(c) $\dfrac{9}{27} = \dfrac{1}{3}$

(d) $\dfrac{45}{66} = \dfrac{15}{22}$

Exercise 5

Set 1

(a) $\dfrac{54}{21} = 2\dfrac{4}{7}$

(b) $\dfrac{90}{75} = 1\dfrac{1}{5}$

(c) $\dfrac{86}{60} = 1\dfrac{13}{30}$

(d) $\dfrac{24}{22} = 1\dfrac{1}{11}$

Set 2

(a) $\dfrac{95}{55} = 1\dfrac{8}{11}$

(b) $\dfrac{18}{13} = 1\dfrac{5}{13}$

(c) $\dfrac{60}{12} = 5$

(d) $\dfrac{26}{5} = 5\dfrac{1}{5}$

Set 3

(a) $\dfrac{68}{17} = 4$

(b) $\dfrac{62}{33} = 1\dfrac{29}{33}$

(c) $\dfrac{99}{27} = 3\dfrac{2}{3}$

(d) $\dfrac{45}{6} = 7\dfrac{1}{2}$

Unit Three
Decimals

A decimal can be thought of as a special way of writing a fraction. Man, having ten fingers, has always found it easiest to classify numbers in terms of units of ten. Decimal fractions continue units of ten in numbers smaller than one. In the United States, we use a decimal system for our money. $4.44 is recognized as four dollars and $\frac{44}{100}$ dollar. A decimal point separates the fractional part from the numbers representing one or more. Because a decimal point is very small, a zero (0) is placed before the fractional part if there are no numbers greater than one. The decimal 0.1 represents one tenth or $\frac{1}{10}$, and the decimal 0.01 represents one hundredth or $\frac{1}{100}$. The number one million *and* one millionth is illustrated in Figure 3-1.

CHANGING DECIMALS INTO FRACTIONS

The way to turn decimal fractions into regular fractions is to make the number(s) to the right of the decimal point the top number (numerator) and to make the bottom number (denominator) a one (1) followed by the same number of zeros (0) as the top number (numerator) has digits. For example, 1.1 becomes $1\frac{1}{10}$ and 4.987654 becomes $4\frac{987654}{1000000}$.

Exercise 6

Try changing the following decimal numbers into fractions. Complete one set of problems, then check your answers at the end of the unit. If you are unable to complete the problems *or* if you complete all the sets but don't score 100% on any set, SEE THE INSTRUCTOR. You *do not* need to complete all the sets *if* you can complete a set with 100% correct and understand the principles.

Set 1	Set 2	Set 3
(a) 1.25 = ?	**(a)** 4.68 = ?	**(a)** 3.65 = ?
(b) 45.3 = ?	**(b)** 36.7 = ?	**(b)** 50.9 = ?
(c) 4.55 = ?	**(c)** 3.36 = ?	**(c)** 5.48 = ?

Work Space

```
1,    0    0    0,    0    0    0    .    0    0    0    0    0    1
m     h    t    t     h    t    u         t    h    t    t    h    m
i     u    e    h     u    e    n         e    u    e    e    u    i
l     n    n    o     n    n    i         n    n    n    n    n    l
l     d    s    u     d    s    t         t    d    t    t    d    l
i     r         s     r         s         h    r    h    h    r    i
o     e         a     e                   s    e    s    s    e    o
n     d         n     d                        d         a    d    n
s                     s                        t              t    t
      t         h     a                        h              h    h
      h         o     n                        s              o    s
      o         u     d                                       u
      u         s     s                                       s
      s         a                                             a
      a         n                                             n
      n         d                                             d
      d         s                                             t
      s                                                       h
                                                              s
```

FIGURE 3-1.
One million AND one millionth

ADDING AND SUBTRACTING DECIMALS

The rule for adding and subtracting decimal numbers is the same rule used for other fractions: use a common bottom number (denominator). The easy way to do this with decimal fractions is to line up the decimal points. To add 1.1 with 20.03 you write it as follows:

$$
\begin{array}{r}
1.1 \\
+20.03 \\
\hline
21.13
\end{array}
$$

1.1 ($1\frac{1}{10}$) is also 1.10 ($1\frac{10}{100}$). When you line up the decimal points, you in essence are changing one tenth to ten hundredths.

Subtraction is performed in the same way. The decimal points are lined up, and, if necessary, zero(s) are added to the top number. For example: $5.3 - 4.02 = ?$

$$
\begin{array}{rcr}
5.3 & & 5.30 \\
-4.02 & \rightarrow & -4.02 \\
\hline
& & 1.28
\end{array}
$$

Exercise 7

Try adding and subtracting the following decimal fractions. Complete one set of problems, then check your answers at the end of the unit. If you are unable to complete the problems *or* if you complete all the sets but don't score 100% on any set, SEE THE INSTRUCTOR. You *do not* need to complete all the sets *if* you can complete a set with 100% correct and understand the principles.

Set 1

(a) $3.45 + 45.2 = ?$
(b) $12.03 + 789.1 = ?$
(c) $3.2 + 45.6 + 30.01 = ?$
(d) $45.03 - 38.1 = ?$
(e) $2.06 - 1.345 = ?$

Set 2

(a) $4.68 + 36.1 = ?$
(b) $89.26 + 48.5 = ?$
(c) $4.6 + 40.5 + 38.04 = ?$
(d) $63.45 - 62.09 = ?$
(e) $5.37 - 4.999 = ?$

Work Space

MULTIPLYING DECIMALS

Decimal numbers can be multiplied like whole numbers with the additional step of placing the decimal point the same number of places to the right in the answer as the decimal point occurs in *both* numbers being multiplied. For example, $0.5 \times 0.5 = 0.25$ ($\frac{1}{2} \times \frac{1}{2} = \frac{1}{4}$). As in regular fractions, if you multiply any number by less than one, the answer is smaller than the original number. Another example is $4.67 \times 3.2 = ?$

$$
\begin{array}{r}
4.67 \\
\times \quad 3.2 \\
\hline
934 \\
1401 \quad \\
\hline
14.944
\end{array}
$$

Exercise 8

Practice multiplying decimals in the following problems. Complete one set of problems, then check your answers at the end of the unit. If you are unable to complete the problems *or* if you complete all the sets but don't score 100% on any set, SEE THE INSTRUCTOR. You *do not* need to complete all the sets *if* you can complete a set with 100% correct and understand the principles.

Work Space

Set 1

(a) $12.3 \times 0.4 = ?$
(b) $1.28 \times 32 = ?$
(c) $4.578 \times 0.365 = ?$

Work Space

Set 2

(a) $12.5 \times 0.3 = ?$
(b) $32.45 \times 46 = ?$
(c) $3.549 \times 42.3 = ?$

Set 3

(a) $15.5 \times 0.7 = ?$
(b) $3.98 \times 56 = ?$
(c) $8.521 \times 1.56 = ?$

DIVIDING DECIMALS

The parts of a division problem are the divisor (number doing the dividing), the dividend (number being divided), and the quotient (answer). The dividend (number being divided) is the same number that would be the top number (numerator) of a fraction, and the divisor (number doing the dividing) is the same as the bottom number (denominator) of a fraction.

$$\frac{\text{dividend (number being divided)}}{\text{divisor (number doing the dividing)}} = \text{quotient (answer)}$$

or

$$\text{divisor (number doing the dividing)} \overline{) \text{dividend (number being divided)}}^{\text{quotient (answer)}}$$

To divide a decimal by a whole number, the decimal point is moved up to the quotient (answer) directly above its placement in the dividend (number being divided). For example:

$$2 \overline{)42.42}^{21.21}$$

Before dividing a decimal or a whole number by a decimal number, the divisor (number doing dividing) must first be turned into a whole number. Earlier it was stated that the top number (numerator) of a fraction and the bottom number (denominator) of a fraction can be multiplied by the same number without changing the fraction. This is the method used for turning the divisor (number doing the dividing) into a whole number. For example:

$$\frac{15.6}{1.2} = \frac{15.6 \times 10}{1.2 \times 10} = \frac{156.0}{12} = 12 \overline{)156}^{13}$$

To multiply by ten, all we have to do is move the decimal point to the right one digit. Therefore, if we move the decimal point the same number of spaces to the right in the divisor (number doing the dividing) and in the dividend (number being divided), we are accomplishing the same thing, only faster. For example:

$$1.2\overline{)15.6} = 12\overline{)156}^{\,13}$$

If necessary, zero(s) are added on the extreme right side of the dividend (number being divided). For example:

$$0.12\overline{)15.6} = 0.12\overline{)15.60}^{\,1\ 30.}$$

Exercise 9

Try decimal division in the following problems. Complete one set of problems, then check your answers at the end of the unit. If you are unable to complete the problems *or* if you complete all the sets but don't score 100% on any set, SEE THE INSTRUCTOR. You *do not* need to complete all the sets *if* you can complete a set with 100% correct and understand the principles.

Set 1

(a) $12.4 \div 0.4 = ?$
(b) $43.2 \div 1.35 = ?$
(c) $215.82 \div 6.54 = ?$
(d) $10.396 \div 0.23 = ?$

Set 2

(a) $36.2 \div 0.4 = ?$
(b) $6.2 \div 1.55 = ?$
(c) $80.016 \div 3.334 = ?$
(d) $2.438 \div 0.23 = ?$

Set 3

(a) $46.4 \div 0.4 = ?$
(b) $70.52 \div 1.64 = ?$
(c) $1.04696 \div 0.023 = ?$
(d) $25.2 \div 0.56 = ?$

Work Space

PERCENT

Percent (or per cent) or % means "in terms of hundredths." In the United States, one cent is one hundredth of one dollar. Earlier you learned that per means "equal." Therefore, percent means "in terms of hundredths of the original." A 70% on a test means you got seventy hundredths of the test correct.

To change a whole or decimal number into a percent, you multiply by 100 in the same way you would change an amount of dollars into an amount of cents (pennies). The easiest way to do this is to move the decimal point two places to the right. Examples:

$$50 = 5000\% \qquad 0.1 = 10\% \qquad 1.125 = 112.5\%$$

To change percents to decimals, you divide by 100 or move the decimal point two places to the left. Remember, the number before the percent sign appears larger. Examples:

$$18\% = 0.18 \qquad 3.4\% = 0.034 \qquad 150\% = 1.5$$

You now know how to change fractions to decimals, and decimals to percents.

☛ **HINTS AND REMINDERS:** The decimal needs to be calculated before converting the decimal to a fraction or a fraction to a decimal.

Exercise 10

Fill in the blank spaces in the following chart. If the percent is filled in, complete the fraction and the decimal. If the decimal is filled in, complete the percent and the fraction. If the fraction is filled in, complete the decimal and the percent.

Fraction	Decimal	Percent
$\frac{1}{4}$		
	0.54	
		20%
		3%
	1.3	
$\frac{6}{25}$		
	7.6	
		0.5%

ROUNDING DECIMALS

When a decimal fraction is obtained by division, it may contain much more accuracy than is wanted or needed. If you are measuring the distance between New York and San Francisco, you don't want it to the millionth of a mile. Use your common sense. Calculate the answer to one more place than needed, then if the last (unnecessary) digit is 5 or more, round the last needed digit up one. If the last unnecessary digit is 4 or less, round the last needed digit down. For example:

(a) 1.333 rounded to hundredths is 1.33
(b) 1.335 rounded to hundredths is 1.34
(c) 1.339 rounded to tenths is 1.3
(d) 1.49999999 rounded to a whole number is 1

A general rule of thumb is to never add more decimal places than were in the original numbers.

Answers to Exercises

Exercise 6

Set 1

(a) $1.25 = 1\frac{25}{100} = 1\frac{1}{4}$

(b) $45.3 = 45\frac{3}{10}$

(c) $4.55 = 4\frac{55}{100} = 4\frac{11}{20}$

Set 2

(a) $4.68 = 4\frac{68}{100} = 4\frac{17}{25}$

(b) $36.7 = 36\frac{7}{10}$

(c) $3.36 = 3\frac{36}{100} = 3\frac{9}{25}$

Set 3

(a) $3.65 = 3\frac{65}{100} = 3\frac{13}{20}$

(b) $50.9 = 50\frac{9}{10}$

(c) $5.48 = 5\frac{48}{100} = 5\frac{12}{25}$

Exercise 7

Set 1

(a) $3.45 + 45.2 = 48.65$
(b) $12.03 + 789.1 = 801.13$
(c) $3.2 + 45.6 + 30.01 = 78.81$
(d) $45.03 - 38.1 = 6.93$
(e) $2.06 - 1.345 = 0.715$

Set 2

(a) $4.68 + 36.1 = 40.78$
(b) $89.26 + 48.5 = 137.76$
(c) $4.6 + 40.5 + 38.04 = 83.14$
(d) $63.45 - 62.09 = 1.36$
(e) $5.37 - 4.999 = 0.371$

Exercise 8

Set 1

(a) $12.3 \times 0.4 = 4.92$
(b) $1.28 \times 32 = 40.96$
(c) $4.578 \times 0.365 = 1.670970$

Set 2

(a) $12.5 \times 0.3 = 3.75$
(b) $32.45 \times 46 = 1492.70$
(c) $3.549 \times 42.3 = 150.1227$

Set 3

(a) $15.5 \times 0.7 = 10.85$
(b) $3.98 \times 56 = 222.88$
(c) $8.521 \times 1.56 = 13.29276$

Exercise 9

Set 1

(a) $12.4 \div 0.4 = 31$
(b) $43.2 \div 1.35 = 32$
(c) $215.82 \div 6.54 = 33$
(d) $10.396 \div 0.23 = 45.23$

Set 2

(a) $36.2 \div 0.4 = 90.5$
(b) $6.2 \div 1.55 = 4$
(c) $80.016 \div 3.334 = 24$
(d) $2.438 \div 0.23 = 10.6$

Set 3

(a) $46.4 \div 0.4 = 116$
(b) $70.52 \div 1.64 = 43$
(c) $1.04696 \div 0.023 = 45.52$
(d) $25.2 \div 0.56 = 45$

Exercise 10

Fraction	Decimal	Percent
$\frac{1}{4}$	0.25	25%
$\frac{27}{50}$	0.54	54%
$\frac{1}{5}$	0.2	20%
$\frac{3}{100}$	0.03	3%
$1\frac{3}{10}$	1.3	103%
$\frac{6}{25}$	0.24	24%
$7\frac{3}{5}$	7.6	760%
$\frac{1}{200}$	0.005	0.5%

Unit Four
Ratio and Proportion

A ratio indicates the relationship of one quantity to another quantity. For example, one ounce of cornflakes contains 110 calories. There is a definite relationship between the weight (or the amount) of the cornflakes and the number of calories (units of heat) they contain. This relationship or ratio can be expressed as:

1) 1 ounce of cornflakes for each 110 calories;
   or
2) 1 ounce of cornflakes per 110 calories;
   or
3) 1 ounce of cornflakes : 110 calories
   or
4) $\dfrac{1 \text{ ounce cornflakes}}{110 \text{ calories}}$
   or
5) 1 ounce cornflakes = 110 calories

A proportion is the expression of the relationship between two ratios. For example, 1 ounce of cornflakes is to 110 calories as 2 ounces of cornflakes are to 220 calories. This can be expressed in writing or in mathematical symbols such as:

1) 1 oz. cornflakes : 110 cal. :: 2 oz. cornflakes : 220 cal.
   or
2) $\dfrac{1 \text{ oz. cornflakes}}{110 \text{ cal.}} = \dfrac{2 \text{ oz. cornflakes}}{220 \text{ cal.}}$

For the rest of this material, the second or fractional method of expressing proportions will be used because it lends itself to mathematical manipulation.

The good news at this point is that you now have been taught all the mathematics you need in order to solve any medication problem. When you learned to multiply, divide, add, and subtract fractions, you also learned to calculate ratio and proportion. And as a nurse you have learned the most basic rule of all: STOP AND THINK BEFORE YOU ACT.

There are two steps to solving a proportional problem. First, isolate the unknown quantity, then do the calculations necessary to reduce the other side of the equation. For example:

$$\frac{?}{4} = \frac{4}{8}$$

First, isolate the ? by multiplying both sides of the equation by four. An equation is a balance, and we can maintain that balance by multiplying each side by the same number or dividing each side by the same number. The new equation looks like this:

$$\frac{4}{1} \times \frac{?}{4} = \frac{4}{8} \times \frac{4}{1}$$

Earlier, the fact that 1 was an automatic bottom number (denominator) was discussed. Because 1 is an automatic bottom number (denominator) and 1 times anything doesn't change the quantity, the proportion can be written as:

$$\frac{4 \times ?}{4} = \frac{4 \times 4}{8}$$

The unknown quantity is isolated when the 4 in the top number (numerator) is divided by the 4 in the bottom number (denominator):

$$\frac{\cancel{4} \times ?}{\cancel{4}} = \frac{4 \times 4}{8}$$

This leaves us with:

$$? = \frac{4 \times 4}{8}$$

From this point, it is a simple calculation to reduce the other side:

$$? = \frac{\overset{1}{\cancel{4}} \times \overset{2}{\cancel{4}}}{\underset{1}{\underset{\cancel{2}}{\cancel{8}}}} = 2$$

A faster way to write it is to multiply both top numbers (numerators) by the bottom number (denominator) of the ratio containing the unknown quantity.

$$\frac{?}{4} = \frac{4}{8} \;\rightarrow\; \frac{4 \times ?}{4} = \frac{\overset{1}{\cancel{4}} \times \overset{2}{\cancel{4}}}{\underset{1}{\underset{\cancel{2}}{\cancel{8}}}} \;\rightarrow\; ? = 2$$

Exercise 11

Try solving for the unknown in the following proportions. Leave your answer in fractional, not decimal form. Complete one set of problems, then check your answers at the end of the unit. If you are unable to complete the problems *or* if you complete all the sets but don't score 100% on any set, SEE THE INSTRUCTOR. You *do not* need to complete all the sets *if* you can complete a set with 100% correct and understand the principles.

Set 1

(a) $\dfrac{?}{2} = \dfrac{5}{10}$

(b) $\dfrac{?}{7} = \dfrac{3}{35}$

(c) $\dfrac{?}{3} = \dfrac{18}{21}$

(d) $\dfrac{5}{4} = \dfrac{?}{36}$

(e) $\dfrac{?}{5} = \dfrac{5}{10}$

(f) $\dfrac{?}{16} = \dfrac{3}{24}$

Set 2

(a) $\dfrac{?}{2} = \dfrac{5}{25}$

(b) $\dfrac{?}{9} = \dfrac{75}{25}$

(c) $\dfrac{?}{3} = \dfrac{5}{25}$

(d) $\dfrac{3}{4} = \dfrac{?}{20}$

(e) $\dfrac{?}{5} = \dfrac{50}{1}$

(f) $\dfrac{?}{11} = \dfrac{75}{25}$

Work Space

Work Space

Set 3

(a) $\dfrac{?}{3} = \dfrac{25}{75}$

(b) $\dfrac{?}{8} = \dfrac{27}{24}$

(c) $\dfrac{?}{7} = \dfrac{25}{75}$

(d) $\dfrac{7}{4} = \dfrac{?}{24}$

(e) $\dfrac{?}{5} = \dfrac{32}{10}$

(f) $\dfrac{?}{26} = \dfrac{27}{24}$

Most medication problems can be set up so that the unknown quantity is in the top number (numerator). If the unknown quantity is in the bottom number (denominator), the steps are still the same. First, isolate the unknown quantity, then reduce the other side of the equation. For example:

$$\frac{3}{?} = \frac{7}{9}$$

Both sides of the equation are multiplied by the unknown quantity:

$$\frac{?}{1} \times \frac{3}{?} = \frac{7}{9} \times \frac{?}{1} \;\rightarrow\; 3 = \frac{7 \times ?}{9}$$

Next, the seven-ninths are removed from the unknown quantity by multiplying each side by nine-sevenths:

$$\frac{9}{7} \times \frac{3}{1} = \frac{7 \times 9 \times ?}{9 \times 7} \;\rightarrow\; \frac{9 \times 3}{7} = ? = \frac{27}{7} = 3\frac{6}{7}$$

Exercise 12

Try working some problems where the unknown is a bottom number (denominator). Leave your answer in fractional, not decimal form. Complete one set of problems, then check your answers at the end of the unit. If you are unable to complete the problems *or* if you complete all the sets but don't score 100% on any set, SEE THE INSTRUCTOR. You *do not* need to complete all the sets *if* you can complete a set with 100% correct and understand the principles.

Set 1

(a) $\dfrac{2}{?} = \dfrac{5}{10}$

(b) $\dfrac{7}{?} = \dfrac{3}{35}$

(c) $\dfrac{3}{?} = \dfrac{18}{21}$

(d) $\dfrac{5}{4} = \dfrac{36}{?}$

(e) $\dfrac{5}{?} = \dfrac{5}{10}$

(f) $\dfrac{16}{?} = \dfrac{3}{24}$

Set 2

(a) $\dfrac{2}{?} = \dfrac{5}{25}$ (c) $\dfrac{3}{?} = \dfrac{5}{25}$ (e) $\dfrac{5}{?} = \dfrac{50}{1}$

(b) $\dfrac{9}{?} = \dfrac{75}{25}$ (d) $\dfrac{3}{4} = \dfrac{20}{?}$ (f) $\dfrac{11}{?} = \dfrac{75}{25}$

Set 3

(a) $\dfrac{5}{?} = \dfrac{25}{75}$ (c) $\dfrac{7}{?} = \dfrac{25}{75}$ (e) $\dfrac{5}{?} = \dfrac{32}{10}$

(b) $\dfrac{3}{?} = \dfrac{27}{24}$ (d) $\dfrac{7}{9} = \dfrac{24}{?}$ (f) $\dfrac{26}{?} = \dfrac{27}{24}$

Work Space

Whenever possible, units of measurement can and should be used in proportional problems. Units of measurement are treated like numbers in that they can be added, subtracted, multiplied, and divided by. Units of measurement serve as a check on the other mathematical processes. For example:

$$\frac{2 \text{ apples}}{5 \text{ children}} = \frac{10 \text{ apples}}{? \text{ children}}$$

In the above equation, the unknown is the number of children there are to 10 apples as 5 children are to 2 apples. The unknown quantity is isolated as follows:

$$\frac{? \times 2 \text{ apples}}{5 \text{ children}} = \frac{10 \text{ apples} \times ?}{? \text{ children}} \rightarrow ? = \frac{10 \text{ apples} \times 5 \text{ children}}{\text{children} \times 2 \text{ apples}}$$

When the unknown is isolated, we can reduce the equation.

$$? = \frac{\overset{5}{\cancel{10 \text{ apples}}} \times 5 \text{ children}}{\cancel{\text{children}} \times \cancel{2 \text{ apples}}} = 25$$

1

The unknown in this case was 25. It was not 25 children because if it were the bottom number (denominator) would read "25 children children" when the answer was substituted for the unknown sign. Normally, the unit of measurement is kept with the symbol representing the unknown in order to avoid confusion. For example, ? children = 25 children.

SETTING UP PROPORTIONS

When setting up proportions from word problems (or medication orders), there is a standard procedure to follow. The first thing to do is to determine what the question asks. As simple as it seems, most mistakes are made by trying to solve a problem prior to reading it. After reading the information, determine what unknown is needed and set up the initial ratio, preferably with the unknown as the top number (numerator). For example:

> There are 110 calories in 1 ounce of cornflakes. How many ounces would a person have to eat for breakfast to consume 1100 calories?

The question is how many ounces (of cornflakes) equal 1100 calories. The initial ratio is:

$$\frac{?\ \text{ounces}}{1100\ \text{calories}}$$

The other side of the equation is the known (110) calories in 1 ounce of cornflakes.* When setting up the second ratio, put the units of measurement in the same location as you did in the initial ratio (i.e., if ounces were in the top number [numerator] in the first ratio, put them in the top number [numerator] in the second ratio). Adding the second ratio establishes the proportion as follows:

$$\frac{?\ \text{ounces}}{1100\ \text{calories}} = \frac{1\ \text{ounce}}{110\ \text{calories}}$$

The unknown is isolated by multiplying both sides by 1100 calories.

$$\frac{?\ \text{ounces} \times 1100\ \text{calories}}{1100\ \text{calories}} = \frac{1\ \text{ounce} \times 1100\ \text{calories}}{110\ \text{calories}}$$

To determine the answer, you just reduce the second ratio.

$$?\ \text{ounces} = \frac{1\ \text{ounce} \times \overset{10}{\cancel{1100}}\ \cancel{\text{calories}}}{\underset{1}{\cancel{110}}\ \cancel{\text{calories}}} = 10\ \text{ounces}$$

Calories are canceled out, leaving the ounces unit of measurement on both sides of the equation. The ounces could of course be canceled by dividing both sides by ounces, leaving ? = 10.

Exercise 13

Try setting up and working the following proportional problems. Complete one set of problems, then check your answers at the end of the unit. If you are unable to complete the problems *or* if you

---

*If there are 110 calories in 1 ounce, there is also 1 ounce in 110 calories.

complete all the sets but don't score 100% on any set, SEE THE INSTRUCTOR. You *do not* need to complete all the sets *if* you can complete a set with 100% correct and understand the principles.

Set 1

(a) There are 25 oranges in each box. How many oranges are there in 24 boxes?

(b) Your car gets 14.2 miles per gallon. How far can you go on 12 gallons of fuel?

(c) There are 20 questions on a test. How many questions were answered correctly if the student earned 90%?

(d) If a teenage girl chews two packs of gum a day, how many packs will she have chewed in 365 days?

(e) If you travel at a constant speed of fifty-five miles per hour, how long will it take you to travel 330 miles?

Set 2

(a) If there are 125 oranges in each box, how many oranges are there in 10 boxes?

(b) Your car gets 14.2 miles per gallon. How far can you go on 14 gallons of fuel?

(c) There are 100 questions on a test. How many questions were answered correctly if the student earned 80%?

(d) If a teenage girl chews two packs of gum a day, how many packs will she have chewed in 40 days?

(e) If you travel at a constant speed of fifty-five miles per hour, how long will it take you to travel 75 miles?

Set 3

(a) There are 25 oranges in each of 100 boxes. How many oranges are there in 24 boxes?

(b) Your car gets 21.2 miles per gallon. How far can you go on 12 gallons of fuel?

(c) There are 30 questions on a test. How many questions were answered correctly if the student earned 90%?

(d) If a teenage girl chews two packs of gum a day, how many packs will she have chewed in 65 days?

(e) If you travel at a constant speed of fifteen miles per hour, how long will it take you to travel 330 miles?

Work Space

Answers to Exercises
Exercise 11

Set 1

(a) $\dfrac{?}{2} = \dfrac{5}{10} \rightarrow ? = \dfrac{2 \times 5}{10} = 1$

(b) $\dfrac{?}{7} = \dfrac{3}{35} \rightarrow ? = \dfrac{3 \times 7}{35} = \dfrac{3}{5}$

(c) $\dfrac{?}{3} = \dfrac{18}{21} = \dfrac{6}{7} \rightarrow ? = \dfrac{6 \times 3}{7} = \dfrac{18}{7} = 2\dfrac{4}{7}$

(d) $\dfrac{5}{4} = \dfrac{?}{36} \rightarrow ? = \dfrac{5 \times 36}{4} = \dfrac{5 \times 9}{1} = 45$

(e) $\dfrac{?}{5} = \dfrac{5}{10} \rightarrow ? = \dfrac{5 \times 5}{10} = 2\dfrac{1}{2}$

(f) $\dfrac{?}{16} = \dfrac{3}{24} \rightarrow ? = \dfrac{3 \times 16}{24} = \dfrac{3 \times 2}{3} = 2$

Set 2

(a) $\dfrac{?}{2} = \dfrac{5}{25} \rightarrow ? = \dfrac{2}{5}$

(b) $\dfrac{?}{9} = \dfrac{75}{25} \rightarrow ? = 27$

(c) $\dfrac{?}{3} = \dfrac{5}{25} \rightarrow ? = \dfrac{3}{5}$

(d) $\dfrac{3}{4} = \dfrac{?}{20} \rightarrow ? = 15$

(e) $\dfrac{?}{5} = \dfrac{50}{1} \rightarrow ? = 250$

(f) $\dfrac{?}{11} = \dfrac{75}{25} \rightarrow ? = 33$

Set 3

(a) $\dfrac{?}{3} = \dfrac{25}{75} \rightarrow ? = 1$

(b) $\dfrac{?}{8} = \dfrac{27}{24} \rightarrow ? = 9$

(c) $\dfrac{?}{7} = \dfrac{25}{75} \rightarrow ? = 2\dfrac{1}{3}$

(d) $\dfrac{7}{4} = \dfrac{?}{24} \rightarrow ? = 42$

(e) $\dfrac{?}{5} = \dfrac{32}{10} \rightarrow ? = 16$

(f) $\dfrac{?}{26} = \dfrac{27}{24} \rightarrow ? = 29\dfrac{1}{4}$

Exercise 12

Set 1

(a) $\dfrac{2}{?} = \dfrac{5}{10} \rightarrow 2 = \dfrac{5 \times ?}{10} \rightarrow ? = \dfrac{2 \times 10}{5} = 4$

(b) $\dfrac{7}{?} = \dfrac{3}{35} \rightarrow 7 = \dfrac{3 \times ?}{35} \rightarrow ? = \dfrac{7 \times 35}{3} = \dfrac{245}{3} = 81\dfrac{2}{3}$

(c) $\dfrac{3}{?} = \dfrac{18}{21} \rightarrow 3 = \dfrac{6 \times ?}{7} \rightarrow ? = \dfrac{7 \times 3}{6} = \dfrac{21}{6} = 3\dfrac{1}{2}$

(d) $\dfrac{5}{4} = \dfrac{36}{?} \rightarrow \dfrac{5 \times ?}{4} = 36 \rightarrow ? = \dfrac{36 \times 4}{5} = \dfrac{144}{5} = 28\dfrac{4}{5}$

(e) $\dfrac{5}{?} = \dfrac{5}{10} \rightarrow 5 = \dfrac{?}{2} \rightarrow ? = 5 \times 2 = 10$

(f) $\dfrac{16}{?} = \dfrac{3}{24} \rightarrow 16 = \dfrac{?}{8} \rightarrow ? = 16 \times 8 = 128$

Set 2

(a) $\dfrac{2}{?} = \dfrac{5}{25} \rightarrow ? = 10$

(b) $\dfrac{9}{?} = \dfrac{75}{25} \rightarrow ? = 3$

Set 3

(a) $\dfrac{5}{?} = \dfrac{25}{75} \rightarrow ? = 15$

(b) $\dfrac{3}{?} = \dfrac{27}{24} \rightarrow ? = 2\dfrac{2}{3}$

(c) $\frac{3}{?} = \frac{5}{25} \rightarrow ? = 15$ **(c)** $\frac{7}{?} = \frac{25}{75} \rightarrow ? = 21$

(d) $\frac{3}{4} = \frac{20}{?} \rightarrow ? = 26\frac{2}{3}$ **(d)** $\frac{7}{9} = \frac{24}{?} \rightarrow ? = 30\frac{6}{7}$

(e) $\frac{5}{?} = \frac{50}{1} \rightarrow ? = \frac{1}{10}$ **(e)** $\frac{5}{?} = \frac{32}{10} \rightarrow ? = 1\frac{9}{16}$

(f) $\frac{11}{?} = \frac{75}{25} \rightarrow ? = 3\frac{2}{3}$ **(f)** $\frac{26}{?} = \frac{27}{24} \rightarrow ? = 23\frac{1}{9}$

Exercise 13

Set 1

(a) There are 25 oranges in each box. How many oranges are there in 24 boxes?

$$\frac{? \text{ oranges}}{24 \text{ boxes}} = \frac{25 \text{ oranges}}{1 \text{ box}} \rightarrow ? \text{ oranges} = \frac{25 \text{ oranges} \times 24 \text{ boxes}}{1 \text{ box}}$$

? oranges = 600 oranges

(b) Your car gets 14.2 miles per gallon. How far can you go on 12 gallons of fuel?

$$\frac{? \text{ miles}}{12 \text{ gal.}} = \frac{14.2 \text{ miles}}{1 \text{ gal.}} \rightarrow ? \text{ miles} = \frac{14.2 \text{ miles} \times 12 \text{ gal.}}{1 \text{ gal.}}$$

? miles = 170.4 miles

(c) There are 20 questions on a test. How many questions were answered correctly if the student earned 90%?

$$\frac{? \text{ questions}}{90\%} = \frac{20 \text{ questions}}{100\%} \rightarrow ? \text{ questions} = \frac{20 \text{ ques.} \times 90\%}{100\%}$$

$$? \text{ questions} = \frac{20 \text{ questions} \times 0.9}{1.00} = 18 \text{ questions}$$

(d) If a teenage girl chews two packs of gum a day, how many packs will she have chewed in 365 days?

$$\frac{? \text{ packs}}{1 \text{ day}} = \frac{2 \text{ packs}}{365 \text{ days}} \rightarrow ? \text{ packs} = \frac{2 \text{ packs} \times 365 \text{ days}}{1 \text{ day}}$$

? packs = 730 packs

(e) If you travel at a constant speed of fifty-five miles per hour, how long will it take you to travel 330 miles?

$$\frac{? \text{ hour}}{330 \text{ miles}} = \frac{1 \text{ hour}}{55 \text{ miles}} \rightarrow ? \text{ hours} = \frac{1 \text{ hour} \times 330 \text{ miles}}{55 \text{ miles}}$$

? hours = 6 hours

Set 2

(a) If there are 125 oranges in each box, how many oranges are there in 10 boxes? <u>1250 oranges</u>

(b) Your car gets 14.2 miles per gallon. How far can you go on 14 gallons of fuel? <u>198.8 miles</u>

(c) There are 100 questions on a test. How many questions were answered correctly if the student earned 80%? <u>80 questions</u>

(d) If a teenage girl chews two packs of gum a day, how many packs will she have chewed in 40 days? <u>80 packs</u>

(e) If you travel at a constant speed of fifty-five miles per hour, how long will it take you to travel 75 miles? $1\frac{4}{11}$ hours

Set 3

(a) There are 25 oranges in each of 100 boxes. How many oranges are there in 24 boxes? <u>6 oranges</u>

(b) Your car gets 21.2 miles per gallon. How far can you go on 12 gallons of fuel? <u>254.4 miles</u>

(c) There are 30 questions on a test. How many questions were answered correctly if the student earned 90%? <u>27 questions</u>

(d) If a teenage girl chews two packs of gum a day, how many packs will she have chewed in 65 days? <u>130 packs</u>

(e) If you travel at a constant speed of fifteen miles per hour, how long will it take you to travel 330 miles? <u>22 hours</u>

Section II
MEDICATIONS

Unit Five
The Metric System

The metric system is subdivided into many different measurement types, three of which are frequently used for medications. The gram is the basic unit of mass,* the liter is the basic unit of capacity, and the meter is the basic unit of length.

UNITS OF LENGTH

One meter is approximately 39.37 inches. The abbreviation for meter is an m. In the metric system, prefixes are used in combination with the basic units to provide units of measurement larger or smaller than the basic unit. One centimeter is one-hundredth of a meter. Therefore, we can say:

$$1 \text{ m} = 100 \text{ cm, and } 100 \text{ cm} = 1 \text{ m}$$

Conversions within the metric system can be done using the ratio and proportion method. For example: "How many centimeters are in 0.5 meter?"
The question provides the ratio:

$$\frac{? \text{ cm}}{0.5 \text{ m}}$$

Mass is similar to weight except for the fact that weight is dependent upon gravity. In outer space you might be weightless, but you would not be massless.

The other side of the proportion is the relationship between centimeters and meters or $\frac{100 \text{ cm}}{1 \text{ m}}$. This provides the proportion:

$$\frac{? \text{ cm}}{0.5 \text{ m}} = \frac{100 \text{ cm}}{1 \text{ m}}$$

cm is then isolated:

$$\frac{0.5 \text{ m}}{1} \times \frac{? \text{ cm}}{0.5 \text{ m}} = \frac{100 \text{ cm}}{1 \text{ m}} \times \frac{0.5 \text{ m}}{1} \rightarrow ? \text{ cm} = \frac{100 \text{ cm}}{1} \times \frac{0.5}{1}$$

Notice how putting in the units enables you to cancel the unit's meter and serves as a check on the proportion. Now we simplify the other side of the equation:

$$? \text{ cm} = 100 \text{ cm} \times 0.5 = 50 \text{ cm}$$

To evaluate the answer, we put it into the original ratio: 50 cm = 0.5 m. Because centimeters are smaller than meters, we can expect more of them and the answer demonstrates this increasing number of smaller units.

An example of converting from centimeters to meters is as follows: "How many meters are in 3 centimeters?"

$$\frac{? \text{ m}}{3 \text{ cm}} = \frac{1 \text{ m}}{100 \text{ cm}} \rightarrow ? \text{ m} = \frac{1 \text{ m} \times 3 \text{ cm}}{100 \text{ cm}} = \frac{3 \text{ m}}{100} = 0.03 \text{ m}$$

In evaluation of the answer 0.03 m = 3 cm, we again see the numbers get bigger as the units get smaller. In the metric system, fractions are usually expressed as decimals.

Other frequently encountered metric length units that consist of a prefix with the word "meter" are:

TABLE 5-1
The Names of the Metric Units of Length

Name	Meter Equivalent	Abbreviation
kilometer	1000 m	km
millimeter	0.001 m	mm
micrometer*	0.000001 m	mcm or μ or μm

One way of visualizing this is:

TABLE 5-2
Metric Units of Length

Kilometer (km)	Meter (m)	Millimeter (mm)	Micrometer (mcm)
1 km	1000 m	1,000,000 mm	1,000,000,000 mcm
0.001 km	1 m	1,000 mm	1,000,000 mcm
0.000001 km	0.001 m	1 mm	1,000 mcm
0.000000001 km	0.000001 m	0.001 mm	1 mcm

The micrometer is frequently called a micron and abbreviated "μ." In pharmacology, the abbreviation of "mcm" is preferred, because a hand written μ can be mistaken for an m.

You need to learn the following equivalents and abbreviations:

1 km = 1000 m
1 m   = 100 cm
1 m   = 1000 mm
1 mm = 1000 mcm

Equivalents or conversion factors can be plugged into a proportional statement because if 1000 m = 1 km, then $\frac{1000 \text{ m}}{1 \text{ km}} = 1$. Any number can be multiplied (or divided) by 1 without changing the quantity represented. Therefore, we can set up a conversion from 5 kilometers to micrometers as follows:

$$\frac{? \text{ mcm}}{5 \text{ km}} = \frac{1000 \text{ m}}{1 \text{ km}} \times \frac{1000 \text{ mm}}{1 \text{ m}} \times \frac{1000 \text{ mcm}}{1 \text{ mm}}$$

The unknown is isolated:

$$? \text{ mcm} = \frac{1000 \text{ m}}{1 \text{ km}} \times \frac{1000 \text{ mm}}{1 \text{ m}} \times \frac{1000 \text{ mcm}}{1 \text{ mm}} \times \frac{5 \text{ km}}{1}$$

After canceling all the units and multiplying, we find:

$$? \text{ mcm} = 5{,}000{,}000{,}000 \text{ mcm}$$

To check we look at 5 km = 5,000,000,000 mcm.
A conversion of 50 cm to kilometers is as follows:

$$\frac{? \text{ km}}{50 \text{ cm}} = \frac{1 \text{ m}}{100 \text{ cm}} \times \frac{1 \text{ km}}{1000 \text{ m}} \rightarrow ? \text{ km} = \frac{1 \text{ m} \times 1 \text{ km} \times 50 \text{ cm}}{100 \text{ cm} \times 1000 \text{ m} \times 1}$$

The units are canceled and the calculations are made, leaving:

$$? \text{ km} = \frac{5 \text{ km}}{10{,}000} = 0.0005 \text{ km}$$

Exercise 14

Find the following equivalents using the ratio and proportion method. It is better to look up the conversion factor(s) than to guess. If you look up a conversion factor while working one set, work the next set. The answers are at the end of the unit.

Set 1   **Work Space**

(a) ? km = 45 m
(b) ? mcm = 340 mm
(c) ? cm = 5 mm
(d) ? mcm = 0.3 m
(e) ? km = 300 cm

Set 2

(a) ? km = 550 m
(b) ? mcm = 0.2 mm
(c) ? cm = 46 mm
(d) ? mcm = 0.0000001 m
(e) ? km = 45 cm

Set 3

(a) ? km = 3 m
(b) ? mcm = 99 mm
(c) ? cm = 542 mm
(d) ? mcm = 5 m
(e) ? km = 5,000 m

UNITS OF CAPACITY

The liter is the basic unit of capacity in the metric system. One liter is approximately equal to 1.057 quarts. The prefixes are the same as those used in units of length and can be visualized as follows:

TABLE 5-3
Metric Units of Capacity

Kiloliter (kl)	Liter (L)	Milliliter (ml)	Microliter (mcl)
1 kl	1000 L	1,000,000 ml	1,000,000,000 mcl
0.001 kl	1 L	1,000 ml	1,000,000 mcl
0.000001 kl	0.001 L	1 ml	1,000 mcl
0.000000001 kl	0.000001 L	0.001 ml	1 mcl

You need to learn the following equivalents and abbreviations:

    1 kl = 1000 L
    1 L   = 1000 ml
    1 ml = 1000 mcl

Two unique factors in units of capacity are (1) the abbreviation "L" is preferable to using the small letter "l" because the letter "l" can be mistaken for the number 1 and (2) cubic centimeter (cc) is used interchangeably with milliliter (i.e., 1 cc = 1 ml and 1 ml = 1 cc).

The conversion of units of capacity measurement occurs in exactly the same manner as the conversion that occurred in dealing with units of length. For example: "How many cc are in one kl?"

$$\frac{? \text{ cc}}{1 \text{ kl}} = \frac{1000 \text{ L}}{1 \text{ kl}} \times \frac{1000 \text{ ml}}{1 \text{ L}} \times \frac{1 \text{ cc}}{1 \text{ ml}} = 1,000,000 \text{ cc}$$

UNITS OF MASS

The gram is the basic unit of mass in the metric system. One gram is approximately equal to 0.035 ounce or the mass of two paper clips. The prefixes are the same as in units of length or capacity and can be visualized as follows:

TABLE 5-4
Metric Units of Mass

Kilogram (kg)	Gram (g)	Milligram (mg)	Microgram (mcg)
1 kg	1000 g	1,000,000 mg	1,000,000,000 mcg
0.001 kg	1 g	1,000 mg	1,000,000 mcg
0.000001 kg	0.001 g	1 mg	1,000 mcg
0.000000001 kg	0.000001 g	0.001 mg	1 mcg

You need to learn the following equivalents and abbreviations:

1 kg = 1000 g or 1000 gm*
1 g = 1000 mg
1 mg = 1000 mcg

The conversion of units of mass measurement occurs in exactly the same manner as the conversion occurred in units of length and in units of capacity. Some drug labels list units of mass in several forms so that conversion isn't necessary, see Figure 5-1.

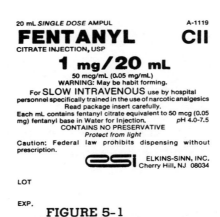

FIGURE 5-1

A drug label with the medication strength listed in both milligrams and micrograms
(Courtesy of Elkins-Sinn, Inc.)

Exercise 15

Try converting these units of mass, length, and capacity. It is better to look up the conversion factor(s) than guess. If you look up a conversion factor in one set, work the next set. The answers are at the end of the unit.

---

*Gram may also be abbreviated gm.

Set 1

(a) ? kl = 32 L
(b) ? mcg = 741 mg
(c) ? cm = 4 mm
(d) ? mcg = 0.9 gm
(e) ? km = 456 cm

Set 2

(a) ? kg = 5.0 g
(b) ? mcg = 0.1 mg
(c) ? cm = 87 mm
(d) ? mcg = 0.0000258 g
(e) ? km = 64 cm

Set 3

(a) ? kl = 7 L
(b) ? mcg = 34 mg
(c) ? cm = 365 mm
(d) ? mcl = 5 L
(e) ? km = 5,999 m

Work Space

Answers to Exercises
Exercise 14

Set 1

(a) 0.045 km = 45 m
(b) 340,000 mcm = 340 mm
(c) 0.5 cm = 5 mm
(d) 300,000 mcm = 0.3 m
(e) 0.003 km = 300 cm

Set 2

(a) 0.550 km = 550 m
(b) 200 mcm = 0.2 mm
(c) 4.6 cm = 46 mm
(d) 0.1 mcm = 0.0000001 m
(e) 0.00045 km = 45 cm

Set 3

(a) 0.003 km = 3 m
(b) 99,000 mcm = 99 mm
(c) 54.2 cm = 542 mm
(d) 5,000,000 mcm = 5 m
(e) 5.000 km = 5,000 m

Exercise 15

Set 1

(a) 0.032 kl = 32 L
(b) 741,000 mcg = 741 mg
(c) 0.4 cm = 4 mm
(d) 900,000 mcg = 0.9 gm
(e) 0.00465 km = 456 cm

Set 2

(a) 0.005 kg = 5.0 g
(b) 100 mcg = 0.1 mg
(c) 8.7 cm = 87 mm
(d) 25.8 mcg = 0.0000258 gm
(e) 0.00064 km = 64 cm

Set 3

(a) 0.007 kl = 7 L
(b) 34,000 mcg = 34 mg
(c) 36.5 cm = 365 mm
(d) 5,000,000 mcl = 5 L
(e) 5.999 km = 5,999 m

Unit Six
Reading Medication Orders

Each medication order or prescription contains seven basic pieces of information: (1) the signature of the person ordering the medication, (2) information to identify the patient, (3) the time the order was written, (4) the medication to be administered, (5) the amount of medication, (6) the route for administration, and (7) the frequency of administration, see Figure 6-1 and Figure 6-2. The usual sequence for the last four items is the name of the medication preceded or followed by the amount of the medication, followed by the route of administration, followed by the frequency of administration.

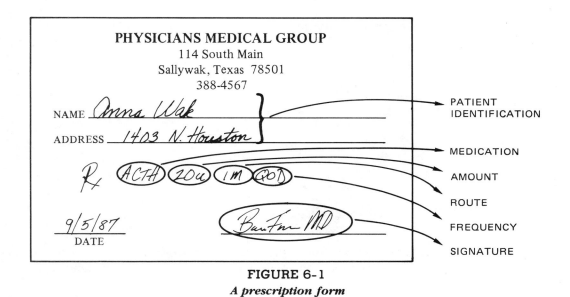

FIGURE 6-1
A prescription form

FIGURE 6-2
A physician's order

MEDICATION AND DOSAGE

The medication and dosage may be preceded by the word "give" or the symbol "Rx" or they may be the first part of the medication order. For example, "ACTH 20 mg," "Rx ACTH 20 mg," and "Give ACTH 20 mg" all mean the same thing. The patient is to receive 20 mg of ACTH.

In the above case, 20 mg is the dosage, so ACTH must be the medication desired. The dosage might be given in terms of mass (i.e., grams), capacity (i.e., ml), length (i.e., cm), or in terms of capsules (caps) or tablets (tabs).

ROUTE OF ADMINISTRATION

Today, medications are administered almost everywhere on and in the body, from behind the ear to directly into the heart. The most common administration routes and their abbreviations are listed.

Route	Abbreviation(s)
Intramuscular	IM
Intravenous	IV
Intradermal	ID
By mouth	p.o.
Sublingual	SL
Subcutaneous	SC or SubQ or SQ
Right Eye	o.d.
Left Eye	o.s.
Both Eyes	o.u.

FREQUENCY OF ADMINISTRATION

Following the route of administration is the indication of when the medication should be given. The following abbreviations are frequently used to indicate the frequency of administration.

Abbreviation(s)	Meaning
stat	Immediately
q.	Every
q.d.	Every day
q.o.d.	Every other day
q.1h	Every hour
q.2h, q.3h, q.4h, etc.	Every 2 hours, Every 3 hours, Every 4 hours, and so forth
h. or hr.	Hour
h.s.	Hour of sleep
b.i.d.	Twice a day
t.i.d.	Three times a day
q.i.d.	Four times a day
p.r.n.	As needed
ad lib.	As desired
a.c.	Before meals
p.c.	After meals

In most cases, periods may or may not be used in the abbreviations, and either capital or small letters may be used.

The time of administration may be followed by additional instructions to the nurse or to the pharmacist.

Exercise 16

Read the following medication orders and write out answers to the questions. After you have answered a set with 100% accuracy, you have completed this unit.

Set 1

The order reads: Polymyxin B Sulfate 10,000 U IV b.i.d.
(a) What amount of medication was ordered?
(b) By what route is the medication to be administered?
(c) When is the medication to be given?
The order reads: Imavate 25 mg p.o. q.i.d.
(d) What amount of medication was ordered?
(e) By what route is the medication to be administered?
(f) When is the medication to be given?

Set 2

The order reads: Deltasone 10 mg p.o. q.d.
(a) What amount of medication was ordered?
(b) By what route is the medication to be administered?
(c) When is the medication to be given?
The order reads: Nalorphine Hydrochloride 0.4 mg IV stat
(d) What amount of medication was ordered?
(e) By what route is the medication to be administered?
(f) When is the medication to be given?

Set 3

The order reads: Chlorprothixene 25 mg IM q.6h
(a) What amount of medication was ordered?
(b) By what route is the medication to be administered?
(c) When is the medication to be given?
The order reads: Phenytoin 100 mg p.o. t.i.d.
(d) What amount of medication was ordered?
(e) By what route is the medication to be administered?
(f) When is the medication to be given?

Work Space

Unit Seven
Dosage Calculation

Calculating medication dosages involves all the steps of the nursing process: assessment and problem identification, planning, implementation, and evaluation.

ASSESSMENT AND PROBLEM IDENTIFICATION

Probably the number one cause of nursing medication mistakes is a failure to properly assess the situation and identify the real problem(s). For example, the physician has ordered 1 cc of Tofranil to be given IM stat to Mrs. S. Tofranil comes as 25 mg per 2 ml. How many ml of Tofranil should you give?

The problem is how many ml are in 1 cc? The other information is not relevant to solving the problem. (If you don't remember the conversion factor from cc to ml, that also becomes part of the problem.)

PLANNING

Plan your dosage calculation strategy to provide the solution to the problem in the simplest way possible. This usually involves placing the unknown quantity in the top number (numerator) on the left-hand side of the equation. For example:

$$\frac{?\ ml}{1\ cc}$$

IMPLEMENTATION

Work neatly and carefully. It takes *much* more time to handle the results of a medication error than it does to do all the calculations neatly.

EVALUATION

Does the answer make sense? A fraction of a capsule is never given. Tablets are seldom divided into portions other than one-half. You will only rarely find a patient getting an injection of less than 0.1 ml or more than 3.0 ml. Look at the equation carefully to see if it appears balanced. Lastly, if you have the slightest doubt that the amount may be wrong, ask someone else to check the calculations prior to administering the medication to a patient.

TABLET DOSAGES

Dosages in tablet form are calculated in the same way as any ratio and proportion problem. For example, the physician wants Mr. G. to receive 650 mg of aspirin. The aspirin tablets available are marked 325 mg/tablet, see Figure 7-1.

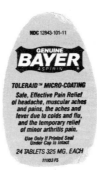

FIGURE 7-1

An aspirin tablet label

(Courtesy of Sterling Drug Incorporated)

Assessment—The problem is "How many tablets contain 650 mg or $\frac{? \text{ tablets}}{650 \text{ mg}}$?"
Planning—You need to compare the ratio of $\frac{? \text{ tablets}}{650 \text{ mg}}$ with $\frac{1 \text{ tablet}}{325 \text{ mg}}$.
Intervention—Work the problem.

$$\frac{? \text{ tablets}}{650 \text{ mg}} = \frac{1 \text{ tablet}}{325 \text{ mg}} \rightarrow ? \text{ tablets} = \frac{1 \text{ tablet} \times \overset{2}{\cancel{650}} \text{ mg}}{\underset{1}{\cancel{325}} \text{ mg}}$$

Therefore, ? tablets = 2 tablets

 WARNING: Be sure to include the units of measurement as a calculation check.

Evaluation—2 tablets is not an unreasonable dose, and $\frac{2 \text{ tablets}}{650 \text{ mg}}$ reduces to $\frac{1 \text{ tablet}}{325 \text{ mg}}$.

Adding Conversion Factors

Conversion factors can be added to the equation the same way they were added in the metric section. For example, the physician orders Ms. A. to receive 1 gram of Tegopen. Tegopen is available in 500 mg tablets.

Assessment—the problem is "How many tablets contain 1 gram?"

Planning—You need to compare $\frac{? \text{ tablets}}{1 \text{ gm}}$ with $\frac{1 \text{ tablet}}{500 \text{ mg}}$ *and* multiply by the grams to milligram conversion factor.

☛ **HINTS AND REMINDERS:** Mg is placed in the top number (numerator) to cancel the mg in the bottom number (denominator).

Implementation—

$$\frac{?\text{ tablets}}{1\text{ gm}} = \frac{1\text{ tablet}}{500\text{ mg}} \times \frac{1000\text{ mg}}{1\text{ gm}} \rightarrow$$

$$?\text{ tablets} = \frac{1\text{ tablet} \times 1000\text{ mg} \times 1\text{ gm}}{\underset{1}{500\text{ mg} \times 1\text{ gm} \times 1}} = 2\text{ tablets}$$

Evaluation—$\frac{2\text{ tablets}}{1\text{ gm}} = \frac{2\text{ tablets}}{1000\text{ mg}} = \frac{1\text{ tablet}}{500\text{ mg}}$, and 2 tablets is not an unreasonable dose.

Exercise 17

Work the following problems. If you complete a set without any mistakes, move on to the next material. If you are unable to complete a set without making mistakes, SEE YOUR INSTRUCTOR. The answers are at the end of the unit.

Set 1

(a) You are to give 64 mg of Thyrar p.o. q.d. The available tablets contain 32 mg. How many tablets do you give?

(b) You need to give Mr. B. 2.5 mg of Methadone Hydrochloride p.o. q.3h p.r.n. Methadone Hydrochloride comes in 5 mg tablets. How many tablets should you give?

(c) The physician has ordered 750 mg Pathocil p.o. q.i.d. for Ms. C. Pathocil comes in 250 mg capsules. How many capsules should she receive?

(d) Mrs. D. is to get 1 gram of Ceclor p.o. each day. How many capsules will she take each day if they are labeled as:

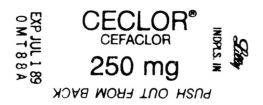

(Courtesy of Eli Lilly and Company)

(e) You are to give Miss E. 75 mg Tofranil p.o. daily. In her medicine tray are tablets labeled Tofranil 50 mg/tablet. How many tablets should you give?

Set 2

(a) You are to give 100 mg of Propacil p.o. q.d. The available tablets contain 50 mg. How many tablets do you give?

(b) You need to give Mr. B. 1.0 gm of Tolinase p.o. q.d. Tolinase comes in 500 mg tablets. How many tablets should you give?

(c) The physician has ordered 750 mg Tegopin p.o. q.6h to Ms. C. Tegopin comes in 250 mg capsules. How many capsules should she receive?

(d) Mrs. D. is to get 60 mg of Pentrobarbital p.o. each day. Pentrobarbital comes in 30 mg capsules. How many will she take each day?

(e) You are to give Miss E. 30 mg Loxitane p.o. b.i.d. In her medicine tray are tablets labeled Loxitane 10 mg/tablet. How many tablets should you give?

Set 3

(a) You are to give 96 mg of Thyrar p.o. q.d. The available tablets contain 32 mg. How many tablets do you give?

(b) You need to give Mr. B. 10 mg of Methadone Hydrochloride p.o. stat. Methadone Hydrochloride comes in 5 mg tablets. How many tablets should you give?

(c) The physician has ordered 0.5 gm Pathocil p.o. t.i.d. for Ms. C. Pathocil comes in 250 mg capsules. How many capsules should she receive?

(d) Mrs. D. is supposed to get 1 gram of Terramycin p.o. each day. Terramycin comes in 125 mg capsules. How many will she take each day?

(e) You are supposed to give Miss E. 75 mg Tofranil p.o. q.d. In her medicine tray are tablets labeled Tofranil 25 mg/tablet. How many tablets should you give?

Work Space

CALCULATION OF LIQUID MEDICATION

Dosage calculation involving liquid medications are the same as calculations involving tablets except the dosage can be more accurately matched to the patient. For example, Jim is supposed to receive 11 mg Seconal Elixir by mouth (p.o.). Seconal Elixir comes 22 mg/5 ml. How many ml should he receive?

Assessment—The problem is the number of ml that equal 11 mg.

Planning—You need to compare ? ml/11 mg with 22 mg/5 ml.

Implementation—

$$\frac{? \text{ ml}}{11 \text{ mg}} = \frac{5 \text{ ml}}{22 \text{ mg}} \rightarrow ? \text{ ml} = \frac{5 \text{ ml} \times \overset{1}{\cancel{11 \text{ mg}}}}{\underset{2}{\cancel{22 \text{ mg}}} \times 1} = \frac{5}{2} \text{ ml} = 2.5 \text{ ml}$$

Evaluation—Two and one-half ml is not an unusual oral medication dose, and 2.5 ml/11 mg is equal to 5 ml/22 mg.

Exercise 18

Work the following problems. If you complete a set without any mistakes, move on to the next material. If you are unable to complete a set without making mistakes, SEE YOUR INSTRUCTOR. The answers are at the end of the unit.

Set 1

(a) You are to give 250 mg of Erythromycin p.o. q.i.d. How many ml do you give from the bottle labeled as:

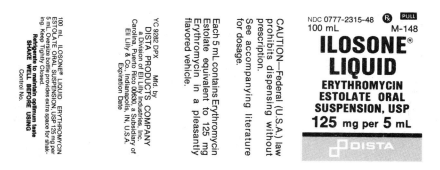

(Courtesy of Dista Products Company)

(b) You need to give Mr. B. 80 mg of Garamycin IM b.i.d. Garamycin comes in 40 mg/cc. How many cc should you give?

(c) The physician has ordered 150 mg Tagamet p.o. q.i.d. for Ms. C. Tagamet comes in 300 mg/ 2 ml. How many ml should she receive?

(d) Mrs. D. is to get 2 mg of Regonol IM each day. Regonol comes in 5 mg per 1 ml. How many ml will she take each day?

(e) You are to give Miss E. 50 mg Benadryl p.o. stat. In her medicine tray is Benadryl labeled 12.5 mg/ 5 ml. How many ml should you give?

Set 2

(a) You are to give 600 mg of Tagamet IM at 8 A.M. The available medication contains 300 mg per ml. How many ml do you give?

(b) You need to give Mr. B. 125 mg of Ilosone p.o. q.i.d. How many ml should you give from the bottle labeled as:

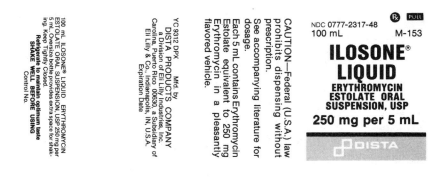

(Courtesy of Dista Products Company)

(c) The physician has ordered 20 mg Benadryl IM q.4h p.r.n. for Ms. C. Benadryl comes in 10 mg/ml. How many ml should she receive?

(d) Mrs. D. is to get 20 mg of Regonal p.o. each day. Regonal comes in 5 mg/1 ml. How many ml will she take each day?

(e) You are to give Miss E. 20 mg Garamycin IM b.i.d. In her medicine tray is Garamycin labeled 40 mg/ml. How many cc should you give?

Set 3

(a) You are to give 100 mg of Seconal p.o. h.s. Seconal is available in 50 mg/ml. How many ml do you give?

(b) You need to give Mr. B. 500 mg of V-Cillin K p.o. t.i.d. V-Cillin K comes in 250 mg/5 cc. How many cc should you give?

(c) The physician has ordered 30 mg Garamycin IM b.i.d. for Ms. C. Garamycin comes in 40 mg per ml. How many ml should she receive?

(d) Mrs. D. is to get 50 mg of Regonal p.o. each day. Regonol comes in 5 mg per 1 cc. How many cc will she take each day?

(e) You are to give Miss E. 150 mg Tagamet IM b.i.d. In her medicine tray is Tagamet labeled 300 mg/2 ml. How many ml should you give?

Work Space

CALCULATION OF RECONSTITUTED DRUGS

Some drugs are unstable in a liquid form, so they are stored in a powder or crystalline form. Prior to administration, the nurse must reconstitute these medications. When working with reconstituted drugs, the nurse must use extreme care in the assessment phase of dosage calculation. Most manufacturers print instructions for reconstituting the medication on either the drug container or on accompanying literature, see Table 7-1.

DO NOT confuse the volume of the liquid you put into the container with the volume of available solution. The volume of available solution is both the volume of the dry drug and the volume of liquid you added. Because you may not be able to withdraw all the medication from the container, and there is a quantity of medication to remain in the hub of the syringe, you may have

TABLE 7-1

Reconstitution of ampicillin (Pollycillin-N) (Reprinted by permission from *Physicians' Desk Reference* © 1986 by Medical Economics Company Inc.)

NDC 0015	Label Claim	Polycillin-N—Reconstitution Volumes		Concentration (in mg/ml)
		Recommended Amount of Diluent	Withdrawable Volume	
7401-20	125 mg	1.2 ml	1.0 ml	125 mg
7402-20	250 mg	1.0 ml	1.0 ml	250 mg
7403-20	500 mg	1.8 ml	2.0 ml	250 mg
7404-20	1.0 gram	3.5 ml	4.0 ml	250 mg
7405-20	2.0 gram	6.8 ml	8.0 ml	250 mg

less solution than the amount of liquid you added. For example, Baby J. is to receive 50 mg of ampicillin IM q.6h. The vial states that you should add 1.2 ml sterile water for a concentration of 125 mg/ml.

Assessment—You need to know how many ml = 50 mg. After adding the 1.2 ml of sterile water, the other ratio will be 1 ml = 125 mg.

Planning—Comparison of ? ml/50 mg and 1 ml/125 mg.

Implementation—

$$\frac{?\ ml}{50\ mg} = \frac{1\ ml}{125\ mg} \rightarrow ?\ ml = \frac{1\ ml \times 50\ \cancel{mg}}{125\ \cancel{mg} \times 1} = \frac{50\ ml}{125} = 0.4\ ml$$

Evaluation—Plugging 0.4 into the equation provides a balanced set of fractions:

$$\frac{0.4\ ml}{50\ mg} = \frac{1\ ml}{125\ mg}$$

Exercise 19

Work the following problems. If you complete a set without any mistakes, move on to the next material. If you are unable to complete a set without making mistakes, SEE YOUR INSTRUCTOR. The answers are at the end of the unit.

Set 1

(a) You are to administer 200 mg ampicillin IM q.4h. How many ml of the solution should you give from a vial mixed according to the following directions?

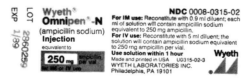

(Courtesy of Wyeth Laboratories)

(b) You are to give 400 mg oxacillin sodium IM q.i.d. The vial states that you should add 2.7 ml of sterile water for injection to the 500 mg vial to produce 250 mg oxacillin sodium per 1.5 ml. How many ml should you administer?

(c) You are to give 660 mg Kefzol IM q.6h. The label states that you should add 2.5 ml of diluent to the 1 gram vial to yield 330 mg/ml. How many ml should you administer?

(d) The patient needs to receive 50 mg Emete-con IM q.3h p.r.n. The label reads, "When reconstituted with 2.2 ml of proper diluent, each vial yields 2 ml of a solution containing 25 mg/ml." How many ml should you give?

(e) You are to administer 1 gram of Staphcillin IM b.i.d. The instructions state, "Add 1.5 ml sterile water for injection to the 1 gram vial. Each 1.0 ml will contain 500 mg of Staphcillin." How many ml should you administer?

Set 2

(a) You are to administer 100 mg ampicillin IM q.4h. The vial states that you should add 1.2 ml of sterile water to provide a concentration of 125 mg/1 ml. How many ml should you administer?

(b) You are to give 250 mg oxacillin sodium IM q.i.d. The vial states that you should add 2.7 ml of sterile water for injection to the 500 mg vial to produce 250 mg of oxacillin sodium per 1.5 ml. How many ml should you give?

(c) You are to give 495 mg Kefzol IM t.i.d. The label states that you should add 2.5 ml diluent to the 1 gram vial to yield 330 mg/ml. How many ml should you give?

(d) The patient needs to receive 25 mg Emete-con IM stat. The label reads, "When reconstituted with 2.2 ml of proper diluent, each vial yields 2 ml of a solution containing 25 mg/ml." How many ml should you administer?

(e) You are to administer 300 mg of Staphcillin IM q.i.d. The instructions state, "Add 1.5 ml of sterile water for injection to the 1 gram vial. Each 1.0 ml will contain 500 mg of Staphcillin." How many ml should you give?

Set 3

(a) You are to administer 300 mg of ampicillin IM q.i.d. The vial states that you should add 1.8 ml of sterile water to provide a concentration of 250 mg/1 ml. How many ml should you give?

(b) You are to give 500 mg oxacillin sodium IM q.6h. The vial states that you should add 2.7 ml of sterile water for injection to the 500 mg vial to produce 250 mg of oxacillin sodium per 1.5 ml. How many ml should you give?

(c) You are to give 165 mg Kefzol IM q.i.d. The label states that you should add 2.5 ml of diluent to the 1 gram vial to yield 330 mg/ml. How many ml should you give?

(d) The patient needs to receive 12.5 mg Emete-con IM stat. The label reads, "When reconstituted with 2.2 ml of proper diluent, each vial yields 2 ml of a solution containing 25 mg/ml." How many ml should be administered?

(e) You are to administer 250 mg of Staphcillin IM t.i.d. The instructions state, "Add 4.7 ml of sterile water for injection to the 4.0 gm vial. Each 1.0 ml will contain 500 mg of Staphcillin." How many ml should you give?

Work Space

CALCULATION OF MEDICATIONS IN UNITS

Some naturally occurring medications are measured in *units*. This group includes some vitamins, some hormones, and some penicillins. The capitol "U" is used as an abbreviation for units. Calculation of these is done with the standard ratio and proportion formula. For example, the physician has ordered 450,000 U Bicillin IM q.d. Bicillin comes in 300,000 U/1 ml. How many ml should you give?

Assessment—The problem is how many ml equals 450,000 U.

Planning—Compare the ratios of ? ml/450,000 U with 1 ml/300,000 U.

Implementation—

$$\frac{? \text{ ml}}{450,000 \text{ U}} = \frac{1 \text{ ml}}{300,000 \text{ U}} \rightarrow ? \text{ ml} = \frac{1 \text{ ml} \times 450,000 \text{ U}}{300,000 \text{ U} \times 1} = 1.5 \text{ ml}$$

Evaluation—1.5 ml is not an excessive injection amount, and the ratios balance

$$\frac{1.5 \text{ ml}}{450,000 \text{ U}} = \frac{1 \text{ ml}}{300,000 \text{ U}}$$

Occasionally, dry medications can be mixed with different amounts of diluent to provide different strengths of the mixed drug. The classic example of this is penicillin G potassium. The label states, "Add 19.6 ml of diluent to provide 50,000 U/ml; add 9.6 ml diluent to provide 100,000 U/ml; add 4.6 ml diluent to provide 200,000 U/ml; add 3.6 ml diluent to provide 250,000 U/ml; add 1.6 ml diluent to provide 500,000 U/ml." The method of reconstitution also appears in related literature, see Figure 7-2.

RECONSTITUTION: 1,000,000 u. vial—add 9.6 ml., 4.6 ml., or 3.6 ml. diluent to provide 100,000 u., 200,000 u., or 250,000 u. per ml., respectively: 5,000,000 u. vial—add 23 ml., 18 ml., 8 ml., or 3 ml. diluent to provide 200,000 u., 250,000 u., 500,000 u., or 1,000,000 u. per ml., respectively. *For I.V. infusion only:* 10,000,000 u. vial—add 15.5 ml. or 5.4 ml. diluent to provide 500,000 u. or 1,000,000 u. per ml., respectively: 20,000,000 u. vial—add 31.6 ml. diluent to provide 500,000 u. per ml.

FIGURE 7-2

Instructions for the reconstitution of Penicillin G Potassium (Reprinted by permission from **Physicians' Desk Reference © 1986 by Medical Economics Company Inc.)**

If you needed to give an adult 400,000 U IM, you would have a wide range of choices to consider in your assessment phase. For an adult, we want to give between 1 and 3 ml. (An infant might require a smaller volume due to smaller muscle mass.) Looking at the choices, we can guess that it will be easier to compare 400,000 to 200,000 than to compare 400,000 to 250,000.

Planning—Comparison of ? ml/400,000 U with 1 ml/200,000.

Implementation—

$$\frac{? \text{ ml}}{400,000 \text{ U}} = \frac{1 \text{ ml}}{200,000 \text{ U}} \rightarrow ? = \frac{1 \text{ ml} \times 400,000 \text{ U}}{200,000 \text{ U} \times 1} = 2 \text{ ml}$$

Evaluation—The ratios balance, and 2 ml is not a proper amount.

🖑 **WARNING:** Any time a vial is mixed that contains more than one dose, the vial needs to be labeled with the date and time of mixing, the amount added, and the nurse's initials.

Exercise 20

Work the following problems. If you complete a set without any mistakes, move on to the next material. If you work all three sets and are unable to answer the final set with 100% correct, SEE THE INSTRUCTOR. The answers are at the end of the unit.

Set 1

(a) You are to give Heparin 7,500 U SC stat. Heparin comes in 5,000 U per ml. How many ml should you give?

(b) You are to give Vitamin E 60 U p.o. q.d. Vitamin E comes in 30 U capsules. How many capsules should you give?

(c) You are to give 60 U ACTH IM q.o.d. ACTH comes in a multiple dose vial containing 40 U/ml. How many ml should you give?

(d) You are to give 150,000 U penicillin G IM q.i.d. The label states, "Add 19.6 ml of diluent to provide 50,000 U/ml; add 9.6 ml diluent to provide 100,000 U/ml; add 4.6 ml diluent to provide 200,000 U/ml; add 3.6 ml diluent to provide 250,000 U/ml; add 1.6 ml diluent to provide 500,000 U/ml." How much will you add, and how many ml will you administer?

(e) You are to give 300,000 U penicillin G IM q.i.d. The label states, "Add 19.6 ml of diluent to provide 50,000 U/ml; add 9.6 ml diluent to provide 100,000 U/ml; add 4.6 ml diluent to provide 200,000 U/ml; add 3.6 ml diluent to provide 250,000 U/ml; add 1.6 ml diluent to provide 500,000 U/ml." How much will you add, and how many ml will you administer?

Set 2

(a) You are to give Heparin 5,000 U SC q.i.d. How many ml should you give from a vial labeled as follows:

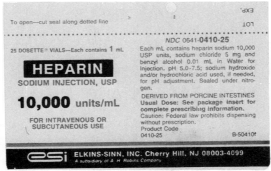

(Courtesy of Elkins-Sinn, Inc.)

(b) You are to give Vitamin E 30 U p.o. q.d. Vitamin E comes in 10 U capsules. How many capsules should you give?

(c) You are to give 60 U ACTH IM q.o.d. ACTH comes in a multiple dose vial containing 80 U/ml. How many ml should you give?

Work Space

(d) You are to give 500,000 U penicillin G IM q.6h. The label states, "Add 19.6 ml of diluent to provide 50,000 U/ml; add 9.6 ml diluent to provide 100,000 U/ml; add 4.6 ml diluent to provide 200,000 U/ml; add 3.6 ml diluent to provide 250,000 U/ml; add 1.6 ml diluent to provide 500,000 U/ml." How much will you add, and how many ml will you administer?

(e) You are to give 30,000 U penicillin G IM q.4h. The label states, "Add 19.6 ml of diluent to provide 50,000 U/ml; add 9.6 ml diluent to provide 100,000 U/ml; add 4.6 ml of diluent to provide 200,000 U/ml; add 3.6 ml of diluent to provide 250,000 U/ml; add 1.6 ml of diluent to provide 500,000 U/ml." How much will you add, and how many ml will you administer?

Set 3

(a) You are to give Heparin 20,000 U SC stat. Heparin comes in 10,000 U per ml. How many ml should you give?

(b) You are to give Vitamin E 20 U p.o. q.d. Vitamin E comes in 10 U capsules. How many capsules should you give?

(c) You are to give 30 U IM q.o.d. ACTH comes in a multiple dose vial containing 40 U/ml. How many ml should you give?

(d) You are to give 600,000 U penicillin G IM b.i.d. The label states, "Add 19.6 ml of diluent to provide 50,000 U/ml; add 9.6 ml diluent to provide 100,000 U/ml; add 4.6 ml diluent to provide 200,000 U/ml; add 3.6 ml diluent to provide 250,000 U/ml; add 1.6 ml diluent to provide 500,000 U/ml." How much will you add, and how many ml will you administer?

(e) You are to give 120,000 U penicillin G IM q.6h. The label states, "Add 19.6 ml of diluent to provide 50,000 U/ml; add 9.6 ml diluent to provide 100,000 U/ml; add 4.6 ml diluent to provide 200,000 U/ml; add 3.6 ml diluent to provide 250,000 U/ml; add 1.6 ml diluent to provide 500,000 U/ml." How much will you add, and how many ml will you administer?

Work Space

Answers to Exercises
Exercise 17

Set 1

(a) 2 tablets
(b) 0.5 tablet
(c) 3 capsules
(d) 4 capsules
(e) 1.5 tablets

Set 2

(a) 2 tablets
(b) 2 tablets
(c) 3 capsules
(d) 2 capsules
(e) 3 tablets

Set 3

(a) 3 tablets
(b) 2 tablets
(c) 2 capsules
(d) 8 capsules
(e) 3 tablets

Exercise 18

Set 1

(a) 10 ml
(b) 2 cc
(c) 1 ml
(d) 0.4 ml
(e) 20 ml

Set 2

(a) 2 ml
(b) 2.5 ml
(c) 2 ml
(d) 4 cc
(e) 0.5 ml

Set 3

(a) 2 ml
(b) 10 cc
(c) 0.75 ml
(d) 10 ml
(e) 1 ml

Exercise 19

Set 1

(a) 0.8 ml
(b) 2.4 ml
(c) 2 ml
(d) 2 ml
(e) 2 ml

Set 2

(a) 0.8 ml
(b) 1.5 ml
(c) 1.5 ml
(d) 1 ml
(e) 0.6 ml

Set 3

(a) 1.2 ml
(b) 3 ml
(c) 0.5 ml
(d) 0.5 ml
(e) 0.5 ml

Exercise 20

Set 1

(a) 1.5 ml
(b) 2 capsules
(c) 1.5 ml
(d) add 9.6 ml
give 1.5 ml
(e) add 4.6 ml
give 1.5 ml

Set 2

(a) 0.5 ml
(b) 3 capsules
(c) 0.75 ml
(d) add 1.6 ml
give 1 ml
(e) add 19.6 ml
give 0.6 ml

Set 3

(a) 2 ml
(b) 2 capsules
(c) 0.75 ml
(d) add 4.6 ml*
give 3 ml
(e) add 9.6 ml
give 1.2 ml

or add 1.6 ml and give 1.2 ml

Section III
OTHER SYSTEMS

Unit Eight
Introduction to the Apothecary System

The apothecary system of measurement is a much older system than the metric system, and originally was based upon the weight of a grain of wheat and the volume of a drop of water. Roman numerals are used in the apothecary system to represent quantities from one-half to one hundred forty. (The numbers we are familiar with are called Hindu-Arabic or Arabic numerals.)

ROMAN NUMERALS

There are six basic Roman Numeral symbols used in medications. They are:

I meaning 1
V meaning 5
X meaning 10
L meaning 50
C meaning 100
ss meaning $\frac{1}{2}$

These symbols may be written in capital or lower case letters and may or may not have a line drawn over them. These symbols are combined to form a number. The following rules describe how they are combined.

First, if a symbol is followed by a symbol (or symbols) with the same or a lower value, the amounts are added to obtain their combined value. For example, VI is 6, XII is 12, XXXIII is 33.

Second, a symbol may be repeated up to three times in succession to form a number. For example, III is 3, XXX is 30, CCC is three hundred.

Third, when a symbol of lower value precedes a symbol of greater value, the amount is the difference between the numbers; for example, IX is 9.

Fourth, when a symbol of lower value is between symbols of greater value, the symbol of lower value is subtracted from the symbol it precedes and the result is added to the number that precedes the lower number. For example, XIV is 14, LIX is 59, and XXXIV is 34.

Last, the least number of symbols is used except that numbers are combined to read like our numbers (the Hindu-Arabic system) in divisions to the left of the decimal point. For example, 15 is XV (not XVX), 55 is LV (not LVX), 46 is XLVI (not VLI), 49 is XLIX (not IL), 99 is XCIX (not IC).

Exercise 21

Write the following Hindu-Arabic numerals in Roman Numerals. The answers are at the end of the unit.

Set 1	Set 2	Set 3
(a) 46	(a) 65	(a) 93
(b) 4	(b) 8	(b) 6
(c) 23	(c) 89	(c) 54
(d) 99	(d) $\frac{1}{2}$	(d) 103
(e) 140	(e) 136	(e) 48

Exercise 22

Write the following Hindu-Arabic numerals in Roman Numerals. The answers are at the end of the unit.

Set 1	Set 2	Set 3
(a) vii	(a) cxl	(a) liv
(b) ss	(b) iv	(b) xiii
(c) xxxiv	(c) xxvi	(c) xxiii
(d) xl	(d) ix	(d) cxxxvi
(e) cv	(e) cii	(e) xc

UNITS OF MEASUREMENT

The predominate unit of weight measurement in the apothecary system is the grain. The abbreviation for grain is gr and sixty grains (gr lx) equal one dram. Dram is abbreviated either dr or with the symbol (ʒ). Eight drams (ʒ viii) equal one ounce. Ounce is abbreviated as oz or with the symbol ʒ.

Minim (abbreviated min or ♏) is the smallest unit of liquid measurement in the apothecary system. Sixty minims (♏ lx) equal one fluid dram (fl ʒ i). Eight fluid drams (fl ʒ viii) equal one fluid ounce (fl ʒ i). Frequently, the fluid designation is omitted.

The apothecary conversion factors you need to learn are:

1 dram (ʒ i)	= 60 grains (gr lx)
1 ounce (ʒ i)	= 8 drams (ʒ viii)
1 fluid dram (ʒ i)	= 60 minims (♏lx)
1 fluid ounce (fl ʒ i)	= 8 fluid drams (fl ʒ viii)

Conversions are calculated using the same ratio and proportion method described in previous sections.

Exercise 23

Work the following conversions within the apothecary system. Remember that Roman Numerals are used for numbers between one-half and 140. The answers are at the end of the unit.

☛ **HINTS AND REMINDERS:** Convert Roman Numerals to Hindu-Arabic numbers for calculations, then back to Roman Numerals to write the answer.

Set 1

(a) fl ʒ ii = ♏ _____
(b) ♏ 240 = fl ʒ _____
(c) ʒ ii = gr _____
(d) gr 960 = ℥ _____
(e) ℥ vi = ʒ _____

Set 2

(a) fl ʒ v = ♏ _____
(b) ♏ 480 = fl ʒ _____
(c) ℥ x = ʒ _____
(d) gr 240 = ʒ _____
(e) ℥ lxiv = ʒ _____

Set 3

(a) fl ʒ ss = ♏ _____
(b) ♏ 60 = fl ʒ _____
(c) ℥ v = ʒ _____
(d) gr 720 = ʒ _____
(e) ℥ ix = gr _____

Answers to Exercises

Exercise 21

Set 1

(a) 46 = xlvi
(b) 4 = iv
(c) 23 = xxiii
(d) 99 = xcix
(e) 140 = cxl

Set 2

(a) 65 = xlv
(b) 8 = viii
(c) 89 = lxxxix
(d) 75 = lxxv
(e) 136 = cxxxvi

Set 3

(a) 93 = xciii
(b) 6 = vi
(c) 54 = liv
(d) 103 = ciii
(e) 48 = xlviii

Exercise 22

Set 1

(a) vii = 7
(b) ss = $\frac{1}{2}$
(c) xxxiv = 34
(d) xl = 40
(e) cv = 105

Set 2

(a) cxl = 140
(b) iv = 4
(c) xxvi = 26
(d) ix = 9
(e) cii = 102

Set 3

(a) liv = 54
(b) xiii = 13
(c) xxiii = 23
(d) cxxxvi = 136
(e) xc = 90

Exercise 23

Set 1

(a) fl ʒ ii = ♏ 960
(b) ♏ 240 = fl ʒ iv
(c) ʒ ii = gr cxx
(d) gr 960 = ℥ ii
(e) ℥ vi = ʒ xlviii

Set 2

(a) fl ʒ v = ♏ 300
(b) ♏ 480 = fl ʒ i
(c) ℥ x = ʒ lxxx
(d) gr 240 = ʒ iv
(e) ℥ lxiv = ʒ vii

Set 3

(a) fl ʒ ss = ♏ xxx
(b) ♏ 60 = fl ʒ i
(c) ℥ v = ʒ xl
(d) gr 720 = ʒ xii
(e) ℥ ix = gr 540

Unit Nine
Apothecary-Metric-Household Conversions

Unfortunately, there is not a single measurement system in use throughout the United States. Efforts have been made to standardize prescriptions using the metric system. These efforts have not been totally successful. At times, the nurse will find a medication labeled in one system and the medication order written in another.

METRIC-APOTHECARY CONVERSIONS

Pharmaceutical companies use exact equivalents when manufacturing medications, but health care workers use approximate (rounded) equivalents in dosage conversion. Conversion factors used in changing between the metric and the apothecary system are NOT exact. 64.79891 mg equals gr i. 64.79891 mg can be rounded to 65 mg if it is rounded to the unit (ones) level. The usual practice is to round this equivalent to 60 mg or round it at the tens level.

The following list contains conversion factors the student needs to learn. When there is a choice of factors, the one given first will be used in these materials.

TABLE 9-1
Metric-Apothecary Conversion Factors

Apothecary	Metric
1 grain (gr i)	60 milligrams (60 mg *or* 65 mg)
15 grains (gr xv *or* gr xvi)	1 gram (1 g)
1 ounce (℥ i)	30 grams (30 g)
15 minims (℥ xv *or* ℥ xvi)	1 millimeter (1 ml)
1 fluid dram (fl ℥ i)	4 millimeters (4 ml)
1 fluid ounce (fl ℥ i)	30 millimeters (30 ml *or* 32 ml)

These conversion factors are used in an equation like all the other conversion factors. For example, the prescription reads A.S.A. gr iv q.4h p.o. p.r.n. The patient needs the A.S.A., but the tablets are marked as 120 mg per tablet. How many tablets should you give? The problem is ? tablets = gr iv.

The proportion you should plan to use in solving the problem is:

$$\frac{?\text{ tablets}}{\text{gr }4} = \frac{1\text{ tablet}}{120\text{ mg}}$$

In working the problem, we come to the point of saying:

$$?\text{ tablets} = \frac{1\text{ tablet} \times \text{gr }4}{120\text{ mg} \times 1}$$

We obviously need some way of canceling the gr in the top number (numerator) and mg in the bottom number (denominator). The way to do that is with the conversion factor 60 mg/gr 1.

$$?\text{ tablets} = \frac{1\text{ tablet} \times \text{gr }4}{120\text{ mg} \times 1} \times \frac{60\text{ mg}}{\text{gr }1} = 2\text{ tablets}$$

To evaluate, we look at whether 2 tablets is an unreasonable amount (it isn't). We can also convert either the grains in the first ratio to milligrams or the milligrams in the second ratio to grains in order to check our proportion.

Because grains are larger than milligrams, and portions of a grain are written in fractions, at times, you may have a fraction in the top number (numerator) and/or the bottom number (denominator). For example, the order reads, "Give atropine 0.5 mg SC stat." The atropine is labeled gr $\frac{1}{120}$/cc. How many cc should you give? The problem is ? cc = 0.5 mg. The plan is to compare ? cc/0.5 mg with 1 cc/gr $\frac{1}{120}$. In implementation we find:

$$?\text{ cc} = \frac{1\text{ cc} \times 0.5\text{ mg}}{\text{gr }\frac{1}{120} \times 1} \times \frac{\text{gr }1}{60\text{ mg}} = \frac{1\text{ cc} \times 0.5}{\frac{1}{120} \times \frac{60}{1}} = \frac{\frac{1}{2}\text{ cc}}{\frac{1}{2}} = 1\text{ cc}$$

In evaluation we find that 1 cc (1 ml) is not an unreasonable dose.

Exercise 24

Work the following problems. If you complete a set without any mistakes, move on to the next material. If you are unable to complete a set without making mistakes, SEE YOUR INSTRUCTOR. The answers are at the end of the unit.

Set 1

(a) The order reads, "Give Morphine gr 1/12 p.o. stat." Morphine comes in 10 mg tablets. How many tablets should you give?

(b) Atropine 0.6 mg SC at 9 A.M. is ordered. It is 8:50 A.M. and you discover the atropine is labeled gr 1/60 per ml. How many ml should you give?

(c) The order reads, "Scopolamine gr 1/300 IM stat." The vial reads Scopolamine 0.2 mg/1 ml. How many ml should you give?

(d) The order reads, "Give U100 insulin 7.5 minims SC p.c." U100 insulin comes in 100 units per ml. How many ml will you be giving?

(e) The order reads, "Give ʒ iv orange juice p.r.n." How many ml of orange juice will you give if the patient needs it?

Set 2

(a) The order reads, "Give Morphine gr 1/3 p.o. p.r.n." Morphine comes in 10 mg tablets. How many tablets should you give?

(b) Atropine 0.6 mg SC at 9 A.M. is ordered. It is 8:50 A.M. and you discover the atropine is labeled gr 1/200 per ml. How many ml should you give?

(c) The order reads, "Scopolamine gr 1/150 IM stat." The vial reads Scopolamine 0.2 mg/1 ml. How many ml should you give?

(d) The order reads, "Give U100 insulin 12 minims SC p.c." U100 insulin comes in 100 units per ml. How many ml will you be giving?

(e) The order reads, "Give ʒ iv orange juice p.r.n." How many ml of orange juice will you give if the patient needs it?

Work Space

HOUSEHOLD MEASUREMENTS-METRIC CONVERSIONS

Occasionally, the nurse has to convert measurements taken in household units into metric units. The following conversion factors apply:

TABLE 9-2
Metric-Household Conversion Factors

Metric	Household
1 kg	2.2 pounds (2.2 lb)
2.5 cm	1 inch (1 in)
4 ml or 5 ml	1 teaspoon (1 tsp)*

Exercise 25

Work the following problems. If you complete a set without any mistakes, move on to the next material. If you are unable to complete a set without making mistakes, SEE YOUR INSTRUCTOR. The answers are at the end of the unit.

Set 1

(a) Baby Bill weighs 6.6 kg. How many pounds does he weigh?
(b) Sally weighs 110 lb. How many kg does she weigh?
(c) Mr. C.'s incision is 2 inches long. How many millimeters long is it?
(d) Ms. D. took 3 teaspoons of Pepto-Bismol. How many cc did she take?

Set 2

(a) Baby Bill weighs 4.6 kg. How many pounds does he weigh?
(b) Sally weighs 88 lb. How many kg does she weigh?
(c) Mr. C.'s incision is 1.5 inches long. How many centimeters long is it?
(d) Ms. D. took 2 teaspoons of Pepto-Bismol. How many cc did she take?

Work Space

---

*In any medication where exact dosage is required, teaspoons should not be used because a household teaspoon may vary from 3 ml to 5 ml.

Answers to Exercises
Exercise 24

Set 1

(a) $\frac{1}{2}$ tablet
(b) 0.6 ml
(c) 1 ml
(d) 0.5 ml
(e) 120 ml

Set 2

(a) 2 tablets
(b) 2 ml
(c) $\frac{1}{2}$ ml
(d) 0.8 ml
(e) 16 ml

Exercise 25

Set 1

(a) 14.52 lb
(b) 50 kg
(c) 100 mm
(d) 12 cc (or 15 cc)

Set 2

(a) 10.12 lb
(b) 40 kg
(c) 3.75 cm
(d) 8 cc (or 10 cc)

Unit Ten
Calculation of IV Flow Rates

Intravenous (IV) fluids are frequently ordered in terms of fluid volume per time period. For example, the physician's order might read "D5W 1000 cc IV q.8h." IV fluids need to be given at a relatively constant rate over the required time span. 1000 cc q.8h DOES NOT mean you can give 1000 cc, then wait eight hours and give another 1000 cc. Special solution administration sets allow nurses to regulate the flow rate. As the IV fluid travels through the administration set, the nurse can see how many drops are falling. By counting the drops that fall each minute, the nurse can tell if the fluid is being administered at the proper rate, and, if necessary, the nurse can adjust the IV administration set to the correct flow rate.

IV fluid flow rates can be calculated using the same ratio and proportion method we used to calculate any other medication. Units of time are used as a measurement system. Fortunately, these units are standardized into days (D.), hours (hr.), minutes (min.), and seconds (sec.). We will also be using a new measurement for liquid amounts. That measurement is drops (gtt), and is NOT the same as minims.

In the case of the D5W ordered at 1000 cc IV q.8h, the problem is how many drops per minute needs to be given, or $\frac{?\,\text{gtt}}{1\,\text{min.}}$.

In this case, the order reads 1000 cc per 8 hr., so, in planning, we have the second half of the proportion.

$$\frac{?\,\text{gtt}}{1\,\text{min.}} = \frac{1000\,\text{cc}}{8\,\text{hr.}}$$

In implementation, we find:

$$?\,\text{gtt} = \frac{1000\,\text{cc} \times 1\,\text{min.}}{8\,\text{hr.} \times 1}$$

Hours and minutes can be canceled by multiplying by 1 hr./60 min. Because 1 hour = 60 minutes, we are multiplying by 1, and multiplying either side by 1 does not change the equation. We now have:

$$? \text{ gtt} = \frac{1000 \text{ cc} \times 1 \text{ min.} \times 1 \text{ hr.}}{8 \text{ hr.} \times 1 \times 60 \text{ min.}}$$

Hours and minutes will cancel, but there is a need to convert cc to drops. The number of drops per cc that a solution administration set delivers is written on the solution administration set box. There are four standard drop rates: 10 drops/cc, 12 drops/cc, 15 drops/cc, and the microdrip set (frequently used for infants and children) that delivers 60 drops/cc. The labels on administration sets give detailed instructions on their use, Figure 10-1.

Directions: Use aseptic technique

The small pore openings of the filter preclude administration through the filter of blood, medications in an emulsion or suspension form or any other medication that is not totally soluble in the carrier solution.

1. Close FLO-TROL® clamp. Prepare and suspend solution container.

2. Remove protector from connector. Insert connector into outlet of solution container. (If using glass container, squeeze drip chamber, insert connector into outlet, suspend container, and release chamber.) Squeeze and release chamber until it is half filled. If solution does not start to flow into filter chamber, squeeze plastic solution container.

3. Remove protector from adapter. Open FLO-TROL clamp. Allow filter to fill. Partially close FLO-TROL clamp. Invert filter housing and tap to remove bubbles. Invert check valve and tap housing to expel air from check valve. Allow filter to hang, fill remainder of set and expel air. **Do not allow air to be trapped in set.**

4. Close FLO-TROL clamp. Attach to venipuncture device. Open clamp and regulate the flow. (10 drops approx. 1 mL)

5. When used for secondary medication, see directions for use with secondary medication set.

Cautions: a) **No restrictions** to flow can be added above the filter. b) **Do not** use this filter set under conditions where pressure greater than 45 psi is generated. c) **Do not** cover or otherwise block the air vent on the filter. d) Puncturing tubing or filter housing can cause air embolism.

For Supplementary Medication: Inject supplementary medication with 20 to 22 gauge needle through the lower injection site with clamp above site closed. **Totally soluble** medication may also be injected through the medication site on solution container. **Use upper injection site with secondary medication set only.** To insure prompt delivery of medication injected into site, be sure that the needle tip projects into the flowing fluid path. **Do not inject supplementary medication into this set when dilution of medication is necessary.**

Notes: a) **Do not** use a regulating clamp above the upper injection site on the CONTINU-FLO® set because of the possibility of air infusion through the secondary medication set. b) To stop flow without disturbing roller adjustment, pull tubing tightly around and beneath small end of clamp. Slide tubing into notch at large end of clamp. c) If fluid path is interrupted, take special precautions to insure fluid path has not been contaminated. d) It is recommended that this device be replaced at least every 48 hours.

Discard after single use.

FIGURE 10-1

Solution administration set label

(Courtesy of Travenol Laboratories, Inc.)

In this case, we will use a 10 drop per cc factor and the equation will become:

$$? \text{ gtt} = \frac{1000 \text{ cc} \times 1 \text{ min.} \times 1 \text{ hr.} \times 10 \text{ gtt}}{8 \text{ hr.} \times 1 \times 60 \text{ min.} \times 1 \text{ cc}}$$

Canceling the units, demonstrates the equation is now equating drops with drops.

$$? \text{ gtt} = \frac{1000 \text{ cc} \times 1 \text{ min.} \times 1 \text{ hr.} \times 10 \text{ gtt}}{8 \text{ hr.} \times 1 \times 60 \text{ min.} \times 1 \text{ cc}}$$

Because there are numerous possible ways to do the mathematical calculations and the student should be proficient with these at this time, just the result will be given.

$$? \text{ gtt} = \frac{1000 \text{ cc} \times 1 \text{ min.} \times 1 \text{ hr.} \times 10 \text{ gtt}}{8 \text{ hr.} \times 1 \times 60 \text{ min.} \times 1 \text{ cc}} = 20.83333333$$

Evaluation—Don't forget to evaluate all your answers. IV flow rates will seldom be less than 10 drops/min. or faster than 80 drops/min. Usual rates are between 15 and 30 drops each minute. 21 drops per minute are within this range.

Drops per minute are rounded off to the nearest whole drop. No human can recognize 0.000003 drop. In this case, since 0.8 is greater than 0.5, the answer is 21 drops.

On occasion, the nurse will have to calculate other information about IVs. For example, if the orders are for 600 cc every 6 hours, the nurse may need to determine how many cc the patient will get each day and what time the next IV bottle (or bag) will need to be started.

In the preceding example, there are two questions. Solve one at a time.

The first problem is how many cc the patient will get each day, or ? cc = 1 day.

In planning the proportion, you must compare ? cc/1 day with 600 cc/6 hr., or

$$\frac{? \text{ cc}}{1 \text{ D.}} = \frac{600 \text{ cc}}{6 \text{ hr.}}$$

In implementation we find:

$$? \text{ cc} = \frac{600 \text{ cc} \times 1 \text{ D.}}{6 \text{ hr.} \times 1}$$

Since one day contains twenty-four hours, we can use that conversion factor.

$$? \text{ cc} = \frac{600 \text{ cc} \times 1 \text{ D.} \times 24 \text{ hr.}}{6 \text{ hr.} \times 1 \quad 1 \text{ D.}}$$

Completing the calculations reveals:

$$? \text{ cc} = \frac{600 \text{ cc} \times 1 \text{ D.} \times 24 \text{ hr.}}{6 \text{ hr.} \times 1 \quad 1 \text{ D.}} = 2400 \text{ cc}$$

Evaluation—Inserting the answer into the original calculation reveals 2400 cc/1 day = 600 cc/6 hr. which is a balanced equation. Some students may be tempted to perform the calculations mentally and omit writing down the formula. These students should be reminded at this point that a patient's health is at risk if they forget to make a single conversion.

The second problem is at what time the next IV bottle should be started. To answer this question, we need to know (assessment) when the present bottle was hung and how much it contained. To restate the problem with the necessary information, the order reads "Give 600 cc D5W q.6h." The present bottle contained 1 L and was started at 10 P.M.

The problem could be stated, "New time = 10 P.M. + ? hr." and "? hr. = 1 L."

The plan to solve the problem would be to compare ? hr./1 L with 6 hr./600 cc.

Implementation would go as follows:

$$? \text{ hr.} = \frac{6 \text{ hr.} \times 1 \text{ L} \times 1000 \text{ cc}}{600 \text{ cc} \times 1 \times 1 \text{ L}} = 10 \text{ hr.}$$

and

New time = 10 P.M. + 10 hr. = 8 A.M.

Evaluation can be as simple as looking at 600 cc every 6 hours and evaluating it with 1000 cc every 10 hours.

Exercise 26

Work the following problems. If you complete a set without any mistakes, move on to the next material. If you are unable to complete a set without making mistakes, SEE YOUR INSTRUCTOR. The answers are at the end of the unit.

Set 1

(a) The physician has ordered 3 L Ringers Lactate IV per day. The solution administration set gives 12 drops per ml. How many ml per minute should drop?

(b) The patient is to receive 500 cc D5W IV in ten hours. The administration set provides 60 drops/ml. How fast will the IV run?

(c) Mr. C. is supposed to get 500 cc of whole blood IV in 3 hours. The blood administration set gives 10 drops per cc. At what rate will the IV run?

(d) Mrs. D. is supposed to receive 1000 cc D5W IV in eight hours. The administration set gives 15 drops per cc. It is now 8 A.M. When will the IV finish?

(e) The physician has ordered 2.1 grams of ampicillin in 1000 cc Normal Saline to run IV every 12 hours. How many mg of ampicillin will the patient get each hour?

Set 2

(a) The physician has ordered 2 L Ringers Lactate IV per day. The solution administration set delivers 12 drops per ml. How many ml per minute should be administered?

(b) The patient is to receive 500 cc D5W in 8 hours. The administration set provides 60 drops/ml. How fast will the IV run?

(c) Mr. C. is supposed to get 500 cc of whole blood in 2 hours. The blood administration set delivers 10 drops per cc. At what rate will the IV run?

(d) Mrs. D. is to receive 1000 cc D5W in eight hours. The administration set delivers 12 drops per cc. It is now 8 A.M. When will the IV finish?

(e) The physician has ordered 2 grams of ampicillin in 1000 cc Normal Saline to run every 10 hours. How many mg of ampicillin will the patient get each hour?

Work Space

Exercise 27

The purpose of this exercise is to challenge your independent thinking skills. Try to solve the following problems using the nursing process and ratio and proportion. The answers and the method of calculation are on page 62. Don't look unless you have solved the problem or have spent at least twenty minutes working on it.

(a) The order reads "Mix 1 gram Ampicillin in 100 cc Normal Saline and give IV at a rate of 50 mg/ 1 minute." The solution administration set delivers 15 drops per cc. How many drops per minute will the IV run at?

(b) You are to give Lidocaine IV at a rate of 2 mg/min. The IV container is labeled, "Lidocaine 1 gm in 1000 ml D5W." The solution administration set delivers 10 gtt/ml. How many drops should fall each minute?

Work Space

Answers to Exercises

Exercise 26

Set 1

(a) 20 gtt/min.
(b) 50 gtt/min.
(c) 28 gtt/min.
(d) 4 P.M.
(e) 175 mg

Set 2

(a) 17 gtt/min.
(b) 63 gtt/min.
(c) 42 gtt/min.
(d) 4 P.M.
(e) 200 mg

Exercise 27

(a) $\dfrac{?\text{ gtt}}{1\text{ min.}} = \dfrac{50\text{ mg}}{1\text{ min.}}$

$$? \text{ gtt} = \frac{50\text{ mg} \times 1\text{ min.} \times 100\text{ cc} \times 1\text{ gm} \times 15\text{ gtt}}{1\text{ min.} \times 1 \qquad 1\text{ gm} \times 1000\text{ mg} \times 1\text{ cc}} = 75\text{ gtt}$$

(b) $\dfrac{?\text{ gtt}}{1\text{ min.}} = \dfrac{2\text{ mg}}{1\text{ min.}} \times \dfrac{1000\text{ ml}}{1\text{ gm}} \times \dfrac{1\text{ gm}}{1000\text{ mg}} \times \dfrac{10\text{ gtt}}{1\text{ ml}} = \dfrac{20\text{ gtt}}{1\text{ min.}}$

Section IV
ADDITIONAL CALCULATIONS

Unit Eleven
Calculation of Infant's and Children's Medications

Infants and children are not just small adults. They differ in metabolism, body surface area, endocrine function, ratio of lean body mass to total body weight, medication absorption, and medication excretion. For these reasons, the U.S. Food and Drug Administration requires special testing of all medications approved for use with pediatric patients.

Each drug has a minimum therapeutic dosage. If an insufficient amount of the drug is given, the desired effect is not obtained. In some cases, such as antibiotics, giving less than the effective amount harms instead of helps the patient. Many drugs also have a toxic dosage; giving too much of these medications harms the patient. The proper dosage is between the minimum therapeutic dosage and the toxic dosage. For an example of dosage instructions, see Table 11-1.

	Oral Loading:	Followed by:	Maintenance:
1. Children 6 months to 9 years	6 mg/kg	4 mg/kg q4h × 3 doses	4 mg/kg q6h
2. Children 9-16 years and young adult smokers	6 mg/kg	3 mg/kg q4h × 3 doses	3 mg/kg q6h
3. Otherwise healthy nonsmoking adults	6 mg/kg	3 mg/kg q6h × 2 doses	3 mg/kg q8h
4. Older patients and patients with cor pulmonale	6 mg/kg	2 mg/kg q6h × 2 doses	2 mg/kg q8h
5. Patients with congestive heart failure	6 mg/kg	2 mg/kg q8h × 2 doses	1–2 mg/kg q12h

TABLE 11-1

Theophylline therapeutic dosages (Reprinted by permission from *Physician's Desk Reference* © 1986 by Medical Economics Company Inc.)

In infants and children, this proper dosage range may vary with the patient's development. It is very important to correctly calculate pediatric dosages and not just estimate a percentage based upon the usual adult dose.

Dosages for adults can also be calculated on the basis of the patient's size. This minimizes side effects and takes into consideration the wide variance in the size of adults. A four-hundred-pound adult has a lot more body than a ninety-pound patient.

DOSAGE BASED UPON WEIGHT

The most common pediatric dosage calculations are based upon the child's weight. This may be in terms of milligrams of medication per pound of body weight or milligrams of medication per kilograms of body mass. For example, the maximum daily dose of Meperidine (Demerol) is 6 mg/kg. The first step to finding the maximum daily dosage for a 20 kg child is to assess the problem as:

$$\frac{? \text{ mg}}{20 \text{ kg}}$$

The nurse then plans to compare that ratio with 6 mg per kg or

$$\frac{? \text{ mg}}{20 \text{ kg}} = \frac{6 \text{ mg}}{1 \text{ kg}}$$

Implementation is fairly simple:

$$\frac{? \text{ mg}}{20 \text{ kg}} = \frac{6 \text{ mg}}{1 \text{ kg}} \times \frac{20 \text{ kg}}{1} = 120 \text{ mg}$$

Evaluation is also simple:

$$\frac{120 \text{ mg}}{20 \text{ kg}} = \frac{6 \text{ mg}}{1 \text{ kg}}$$

If the child's weight is in pounds and the dosage is in kilograms, we merely multiply by the conversion factor of 2.2 pounds = 1 kilogram. For example, the maximum daily dosage for Meperidine is 6 mg/kg and the child's weight is 33 pounds. The assessment is the same:

$$\frac{? \text{ mg}}{33 \text{ lb}}$$

Planning is the same except for multiplying by the conversion factor:

$$\frac{? \text{ mg}}{33 \text{ lb}} = \frac{6 \text{ mg}}{1 \text{ kg}} \times \frac{1 \text{ kg}}{2.2 \text{ lb}}$$

Implementation is essentially the same:

$$\frac{? \text{ mg}}{33 \text{ lb}} = \frac{6 \text{ mg}}{1 \text{ kg}} \times \frac{1 \text{ kg}}{2.2 \text{ lb}} \times \frac{33 \text{ lb}}{1} = \frac{198 \text{ mg}}{2.2} = 90 \text{ mg}$$

Evaluation can be made easier by substituting 2.2 lb for the 1 kg.

$$\frac{90 \text{ mg}}{20 \text{ lb}} = \frac{6 \text{ mg}}{2.2 \text{ lb}}$$

CALCULATING INDIVIDUAL DOSES

Frequently in pediatrics, the dosages are given in terms of a daily dose that is divided into 2 to 6 individual doses. For example, the dose of Meperidine was a maximum of 6 mg/kg/day. If the 20 kg child was getting a dose of Meperidine every 4 hours, we would need to know the maximum dose every four hours.

The assessment of the problem would be "How many mg per 20 kg per 4 hours?" or:

$$\frac{\dfrac{?\text{ mg}}{20\text{ kg}}}{4\text{ hr.}}$$

In planning, ? mg/20 kg/4 hr needs to be compared with 6 mg/1 kg/day, or:

$$\frac{\dfrac{?\text{ mg}}{20\text{ kg}}}{4\text{ hr.}} = \frac{\dfrac{6\text{ mg}}{1\text{ kg}}}{1\text{ day}}$$

In the implementation step, 1 day is divided by one to permit it to be inverted and multiplied. Both sides are multiplied by 4 hr. to clear the bottom number (denominator) of the left fraction. The equation now looks like this:

$$\frac{4\text{ hr.}}{1} \times \frac{\dfrac{?\text{ mg}}{20\text{ kg}}}{4\text{ hr.}} = \frac{6\text{ mg}}{1\text{ kg}} \times \frac{1}{1\text{ day}} \times \frac{4\text{ hr.}}{1}$$

4 hr. in the left ratio cancels, leaving:

$$\frac{?\text{ mg}}{20\text{ kg}} = \frac{6\text{ mg}}{1\text{ kg}} \times \frac{1}{1\text{ day}} \times \frac{4\text{ hr.}}{1}$$

Both sides are then multiplied by 20 kg to cancel the left ratio bottom number (denominator), and the right side ratio is multiplied by the conversion factor 1 day/24 hr. to yield:

$$\frac{20\text{ kg}}{1} \times \frac{?\text{ mg}}{20\text{ kg}} = \frac{6\text{ mg}}{1\text{ kg}} \times \frac{1}{1\text{ day}} \times \frac{4\text{ hr.}}{1} \times \frac{20\text{ kg}}{1} \times \frac{1\text{ day}}{24\text{ hr.}}$$

After all the cancellations are finished, we have:

$$\frac{\cancel{20\text{ kg}}}{1} \times \frac{?\text{ mg}}{\cancel{20\text{ kg}}} = \frac{\overset{1}{\cancel{6}}\text{ mg}}{1\ \cancel{\text{kg}}} \times \frac{1}{1\ \cancel{\text{day}}} \times \frac{\overset{1}{\cancel{4\text{ hr.}}}}{1} \times \frac{20\ \cancel{\text{kg}}}{1} \times \frac{1\ \cancel{\text{day}}}{\underset{\underset{1}{6}}{\cancel{24\text{ hr.}}}}$$

or

$$?\text{ mg} = 20\text{ mg}$$

In evaluation we find:

$$\frac{\dfrac{20\text{ mg}}{20\text{ kg}}}{4\text{ hr.}} = \frac{\dfrac{6\text{ mg}}{1\text{ kg}}}{1\text{ day}}$$

1 mg/1 kg/4 hr. is the same as 6 mg/1 kg/24 hr.

Exercise 28

The answers to the following problems are located at the end of this unit. Complete one set of problems, then check your answers. If you are unable to complete the problems, *or* if you complete all the sets without being able to score 100% on any set, SEE THE INSTRUCTOR. You *do not* need to complete all the sets *if* you can complete a set with 100% correct and understand the principles.

Set 1

(a) The child weighs 30 kg, and is supposed to get Gantrisin IM. The pediatric dose of Gantrisin is 60 mg/kg/day divided into two doses daily. How much should this child receive in each dose?

(b) The child weighs 32 kg, and is supposed to receive Amobarbital sodium p.o. at gr 1/10 per kg per dose. How many grains should the child receive?

(c) The patient is supposed to receive Pseudoephedrine p.o. at 4 mg/kg/day. The patient weighs 26 kg, and is supposed to receive 4 equal doses each day. How much Pseudoephedrine should the patient receive in each dose?

(d) The child is supposed to receive Oxacillin IM at a rate of 25 mg/lb/day in equally divided doses at six hour intervals. The child weighs 26 pounds. How much should be in each dose?

(e) The child weighs 44 pounds, and is supposed to receive Colase IM at a rate of 4 mg/kg/day in three equally divided doses. How much would be in each dose?

Set 2

(a) The child is supposed to receive Heparin SC at a rate of 0.5 mg/kg per dose. The child weighs 10 kg. How much should be given in the dose?

(b) The patient weighs 22 kg. This patient is supposed to receive Ampicillin p.o. 50 mg/kg/day in equal doses given every six hours. How many milligrams should be in each dose?

(c) The child is supposed to receive 15 mg/kg/day of Kanamycin IM in equal doses given every 12 hours. The child weighs 11 pounds. How much should she receive in each dose?

(d) The child weighs 22 kg, and is supposed to get Gantrisin IM. The pediatric dose of Gantrisin is 60 mg/kg/day divided into two doses daily. How much should this child receive in each dose?

(e) The child weighs 11 kg and is supposed to receive Amobarbital sodium IM at gr 1/10 per kg per dose. How many grains should the child receive?

Set 3

(a) The patient is supposed to receive Pseudoephedrine p.o. at 4 mg/kg/day. The patient weighs 22 kg, and is supposed to receive 4 equal doses each day. How much Pseudoephedrine should the patient receive in each dose?

(b) The child is supposed to receive Oxacillin IM at a rate of 25 mg/lb/day in equally divided doses at six hour intervals. The child weighs 56 pounds. How much should be in each dose?

(c) The child weighs 22 pounds and is supposed to receive Colase IM at a rate of 4 mg/kg/day in three equally divided doses. How much would be in each dose?

(d) The child is supposed to receive Heparin SC at a rate of 0.5 mg/kg per dose. The child weighs 15 kg. How much should be given in the dose?

(e) The patient weighs 28 kg. This patient is supposed to receive Ampicillin p.o. 50 mg/kg/day in equal doses given every six hours. How many milligrams should be in each dose?

Work Space

CHECKING PRESCRIBED DOSES

Nurses seldom have to calculate doses based upon milligrams per kilograms. They do, however, frequently have to check prescribed doses to see if they are under the toxic amount and over the minimum therapeutic dosage. The nurse could calculate both the toxic dosage and the minimum therapeutic dosage to see where the prescribed dosage falls. An easier method is to calculate how many milligrams the patient receives for each kilogram of body weight and to compare that figure to the minimum and maximum doses. If the prescription calls for too much or too little medication, the individual prescribing the medication should be notified.

For example, the physician ordered Ampicillin 250 mg IM q.6h. The patient weighs 10 kg. The range for Ampicillin is 25 mg/kg/day to 200 mg/kg/day.

Assessment—This time we need to find out how many mg/1 kg/1 day, or:

$$\frac{\frac{? \text{ mg}}{1 \text{ kg}}}{1 \text{ day}}$$

Planning—? mg/kg/day needs to be compared with the prescribed dose of 250 mg/10 kg/ 6 hr., or:

$$\frac{\frac{? \text{ mg}}{1 \text{ kg}}}{1 \text{ day}} = \frac{250 \text{ mg}}{\frac{10 \text{ kg}}{6 \text{ hr.}}}$$

Implementation—The same process is followed as was discussed earlier in this section:

$$? \text{ mg} = \frac{250 \text{ mg}}{10 \text{ kg}} \times \frac{1}{6 \text{ hr.}} \times \frac{1 \text{ day}}{1} \times \frac{1 \text{ kg}}{1} \times \frac{24 \text{ hr.}}{1 \text{ day}}$$

Canceling, we find:

$$? \text{ mg} = \frac{250 \text{ mg}}{10 \text{ kg}} \times \frac{1}{6 \text{ hr.}} \times \frac{1 \text{ day}}{1} \times \frac{1 \text{ kg}}{1} \times \frac{\overset{4}{24 \text{ hr.}}}{1 \text{ day}} = 100 \text{ mg}$$

Evaluation—100 mg/kg/day is within the range of 25 to 200 mg/kg/day.

CALCULATIONS BASED UPON BODY SURFACE AREA

At times, pediatric medications are calculated based upon body surface area (BSA). BSA is measured in terms of square meters (m^2). A child's BSA is determined by taking the child's height and weight and using these as reference points on a *nomogram*. An example of a nomogram is located in Figure 11-1. To read a nomogram, you place a straight line from the child's weight to the child's height. BSA is indicated by where the line crosses the surface area column. For example, a newborn weighing 8.5 pounds (8 lb and 8 oz) with a height of 21 inches would have a BSA of 0.25 m^2.

BSA is used in formulas calling for mg/m^2 in exactly the same way weight is used in formulas calling for mg/kg. For example, the child's height is 36 inches and weight is 30 pounds. The child is to get a dose of Dimenhydrinate 37.5 mg/m^2.

Assessment—Based upon BSA obtained from the nomogram:

$$\frac{? \text{ mg}}{0.6 \text{ m}^2}$$

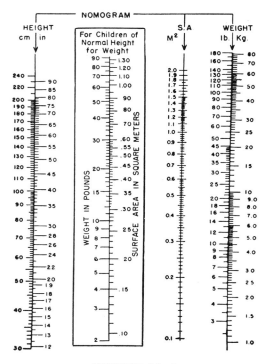

FIGURE 11-1

A nomogram for the estimation of body surface area. (Reprinted from Behrman, R.E. and Vaughan, V.C. Nelson Textbook of Pediatrics, 12th Ed., 1983, with permission from W.B. Saunders Company, Philadelphia, PA 19105 and R.E. Behrman, MD, Case Western Reserve University, School of Medicine, Cleveland, OH 44106.)

Planning—

$$\frac{?\ mg}{0.6\ m^2} = \frac{37.5\ mg}{1\ m^2}$$

Implementation—

$$?\ mg = \frac{37.5\ mg}{1\ m^2} \times \frac{0.6\ m^2}{1} = 22.5\ mg$$

Evaluation—

$$\frac{22.5\ mg}{0.6\ m^2} = \frac{37.5\ mg}{1\ m^2}$$

CHILD'S DOSE AS A PROPORTION OF ADULT'S DOSE

Clark's rule provides a method of calculating a child's dose based upon the adult dose.

WARNING: This rule should not be used unless the drug reference states the child's dosage is proportionate to the adult dosage.

The rule states that the adult dose is based upon a 150 pound adult, therefore:

$$child's\ dose = \frac{child's\ weight}{150\ lb} \times adult\ dose$$

For example, the *Physicians' Desk Reference* (PDR) states that the digitalization dose of Lanoxin for a child 10 years and over is based upon adult doses in proportion to their body weight. If an 11-year-old weighs 100 pounds and the adult dose is 1.0 mg, the formula would be:

$$? \text{ mg} = \frac{100 \text{ lb}}{150 \text{ lb}} \times 1.0 \text{ mg} = 0.7 \text{ mg}$$

Try applying Clark's rule, BSA, and checking prescribed doses in the following problems.

Exercise 29

The answers to the following problems are located at the end of this unit. Complete one set of problems, then check your answers. If you are unable to complete the problems, or if you complete all the sets but don't score 100% on any set, SEE THE INSTRUCTOR. You *do not* need to complete all the sets *if* you can complete a set with 100% correct and understand the principles.

Set 1

(a) A child weighs 40 kg and is supposed to get Kefzol 200 mg IM q.6h. The range for Kefzol is 25 mg to 100 mg/kg/day. Is this amount within that range?

(b) A child weighs 34 kg and is supposed to receive Prostaphlin 100 mg IM q.6h. The dosage range for Prostaphlin is 50 mg to 100 mg/kg/day. Is this amount within that range?

(c) A child is 90 cm tall and weighs 10 kg. This individual is supposed to receive Dilantin p.o. at a rate of 250 mg/m². How much Dilantin should she receive?

(d) A child is 35 inches tall and weighs 50 pounds. This child is supposed to receive Benadryl p.o. at a rate of 150 mg/m²/24 hr., divided into equal doses given every eight hours. How much will this child receive in each dose?

(e) A 12-year-old child weighs 120 lb and is supposed to receive a proportional dose of Lanoxin p.o. The adult dose of Lanoxin is 1.0 mg. How much should this child receive?

Set 2

(a) A child weighs 20 kg and is supposed to get Kefzol 500 mg IM q.6h. The range for Kefzol is 25 mg to 100 mg/kg/day. Is this amount within that range?

(b) A child weighs 54 kg and is supposed to receive Prostaphlin 1000 mg IM q.6h. The dosage range for Prostaphlin is 50 mg to 100 mg/kg/day. Is this amount within that range?

(c) A child is 80 cm tall and weighs 20 kg. This individual is supposed to receive Dilantin p.o. at a rate of 250 mg/m². How much Dilantin should the child receive?

(d) A child is 40 inches tall and weighs 60 pounds. This child is supposed to receive Benadryl p.o. at a rate of 150 mg/m²/24 hr. divided into equal doses given every eight hours. How much will this child receive in each dose?

(e) A 10-year-old child weighs 75 lb and is supposed to receive a proportional dose of Lanoxin p.o. The adult dose of Lanoxin is 1.0 mg. How much should this child receive?

Work Space

Answers to Exercises
Exercise 28

Set 1

(a) 900 mg
(b) gr 3 1/5
(c) 26 mg
(d) 162.5 mg
(e) 27 mg (or 26.7)

Set 2

(a) 5 mg
(b) 275 mg
(c) 37.5 mg
(d) 660 mg
(e) gr 1 1/10

Set 3

(a) 22 mg
(b) 350 mg
(c) 13.3 mg
(d) 7.5 mg
(e) 350 mg

Exercise 29

Set 1

(a) 20 mg/kg/day TOO LITTLE
(b) 12 mg/kg/day TOO LITTLE
(c) 125 mg
(d) 40 mg
(e) 0.8 mg

Set 2

(a) 100 mg/kg/day O.K.
(b) 74 mg/kg/day O.K.
(c) 175 mg
(d) 45 mg
(e) 0.5 mg

Unit Twelve
Miscellaneous Calculations

TEMPERATURE CONVERSIONS

Temperature is commonly recorded in either degrees Fahrenheit or degrees Celsius (Celsius degrees are also referred to as Centigrade degrees). In about 1700 A.D., a Northern European instrument maker named Fahrenheit built one of the first accurate thermometers. Because there was no established temperature scale, he mixed equal weights of salt and water and used the temperature of that mixture as zero degrees (0°). The top of his scale was measured by holding the thermometer in a human hand. He subdivided his scale into units of eight, so the top became 96°.

A few years later, an instrument maker named Celsius developed his own scale to compete with Mr. Fahrenheit's thermometers. Mr. Celsius based his scale upon the freezing point and boiling point of pure water at sea level. The freezing point he designated as zero degrees (0°C) and the boiling point as one hundred degrees (100°C). His scale became known as the centigrade scale because it is based upon 100 degrees. It is fortunate that both centigrade and Celsius start with the letter "C" because the scale is known by both names, but it is abbreviated as C.

The conversion factor for degrees Fahrenheit to degrees Celsius (Centigrade) is °F−32° = 1.8 × °C. The only tricky point in using this formula is to remember when to subtract the 32°. Deal with the known side of the equation first. When converting from degrees Fahrenheit to degrees Celsius, the 32° are subtracted first, because you know the number of Fahrenheit degrees.

For example, to convert 98.6°F to °C, the following process is used:

$$98.6°F - 32° = 1.8 \times ?°C$$

$$66.6° = 1.8 \times ?°C$$

Next, 1.8 is removed from the Celsius side by dividing both sides by 1.8.

$$\frac{66.2°}{1.8} = \frac{1.8 \times ?°C}{1.8}$$

$$37° = ?°C$$

In converting from Celsius to Fahrenheit, the first step is multiplication. For example, figure how many degrees Fahrenheit is 98.6 degrees Celsius:

$$?°F - 32° = 1.8 \times 98.6°C$$

$$?°F - 32° = 177.48°$$

32° is removed from the Fahrenheit side by adding it to both sides.

$$?°F - 32° + 32° = 177.48° + 32°$$

$$?°F = 209.48°$$

Temperature conversions should be rounded to the same decimal place as the original number. In this case 209.48 would be rounded to 209.5. This tells the reader the original degree of accuracy. Health care workers have developed the practice of rounding to the even tenth of a degree when measuring body temperature. (This is because glass thermometers are accurate to the even tenth of a degree.) If 209.48 were a body temperature, it would round to 209.4°.

Evaluation of these conversions can be done by comparing the calculation results with some known Fahrenheit-Celsius equivalents, Table 12-1.

TABLE 12-1
Fahrenheit-Celsius Equivalents

	Fahrenheit	**Celsius**
freezing of water	32°	0°
normal human oral temperature	98.6°	37°
boiling of water	212°	100°

The result of 209.5°F = 98.6°C is fairly close to the boiling point of water. Both amounts are slightly less than the boiling point, so the answer appears to be reasonable.

Exercise 30

The answers to the following problems are located at the end of this unit. Complete one set of problems, then check your answers. If you are unable to complete the problems *or* if you complete all the sets but don't score 100% on any set, SEE THE INSTRUCTOR. You *do not* need to complete all the sets *if* you can complete a set with 100% correct and understand the principles.

Set 1   **Work Space**

(a) $?°F = 32.0°C$
(b) $?°F = 101°C$
(c) $?°F = 3.4°C$
(d) $99.2°F = ?°C$
(e) $58°F = ?°C$
(f) $3.02°F = ?°C$

Set 2   **Work Space**

(a) ?°F = 45.0°C
(b) ?°F = 105°C
(c) ?°F = 4.6°C
(d) 99.8°F = ?°C
(e) 70.0°F = ?°C
(f) 4.16°F = ?°C

Set 3

(a) ?°F = 36.0°C
(b) ?°F = 110°C
(c) ?°F = 2.1°C
(d) 92.4°F = ?°C
(e) 60°F = ?°C
(f) 3.28°F = ?°C

STRENGTH OF SOLUTIONS—WEIGHT/VOLUME

The strength of a given solution can be described in several different fashions. In calculating medications, you used the weight of the medication in relation to the volume of the medication (i.e., 2.5 mg/1 ml), see Figure 12-1. The colon (:) may be used instead of the slash mark (/) to indicate division. Therefore, 2.5 mg per ml may be written 2.5 mg:1 ml.

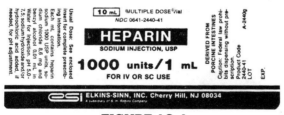

FIGURE 12-1

A label showing the relationship of weight to volume in a medication
(Courtesy of Elkins-Sinn, Inc.)

Grams percent (gm %) is also termed percent (%) and is based upon one gram per one hundred milliliters, see Figure 12-2. A fifty percent solution would then have fifty grams of the solid material for each one hundred milliliters of liquid, or (50% = 50 gm/100 ml). To calculate the percentage, we need to compute the number of grams per 100 ml. The ratio and proportion method can be used. For example, to convert 2.5 milligrams per milliliter to percent:

$$\frac{?\ gm}{100\ ml} = \frac{2.5\ mg}{1\ ml} \rightarrow ?\ gm = \frac{2.5\ mg}{1\ ml} \times \frac{100\ ml}{1} \times \frac{1\ gm}{1000\ mg}$$

$$?\ gm = 0.25\ gm = 0.25\%$$

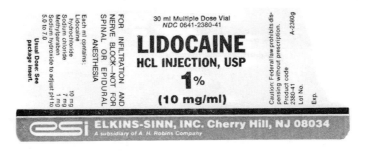

FIGURE 12-2
A label showing grams percent of a medication
(Courtesy of Elkins-Sinn, Inc.)

A variation of this process can be used to determine the amount (in weight) of a chemical that needs to be added to a solution in order to provide a given percentage concentration. For example, if you needed to make 1 liter of physiologic (normal) saline, and you knew Normal Saline was 0.9% NaCl:

$$\frac{? \text{ gm}}{1 \text{ L}} = \frac{0.9 \text{ gm}}{100 \text{ ml}}$$

$$? \text{ gm} = \frac{0.9 \text{ gm}}{100 \text{ ml}} \times \frac{1 \text{ L}}{1} \times \frac{1000 \text{ ml}}{1 \text{ L}} = 9 \text{ gm}$$

A different method of describing the strength of a solution is in terms of grams per milliliter. This method uses the colon to describe the relationship, but the units of measurement are not used. The number preceding the colon indicates the weight of the substance in grams, and the number following the colon indicates the amount of solution. For example, 1:100 means 1 gram per 100 ml.

A last method for describing the relation of solids to a liquid is milliequivalents (mEq). The number of milliequivalents is determined by taking the molecular weight (sum of the atomic weights of each atom in the molecule) divided by the valence of the molecule in order to yield the equivalent weight. The total weight of the molecules expressed in milligrams is divided by the equivalent weight to provide the number of milliequivalents. For example, KCl has a molecular weight of 75 and a valence of 1, yielding an equivalent weight of 75. 150 mg of KCl would then be equal to 2 mEq KCl.

Fortunately, nurses seldom have to calculate mEq. Nurses do have to use mEq in calculations when the ratio of mEq per volume is given. In this case, mEq are treated as any other unit of measurement. For example, the nurse needs to add 10 mEq KCl to 1000 ml IV fluid. KCl comes in 20 mEq per 15 ml. How many ml should be added?

$$\frac{? \text{ ml}}{10 \text{ mEq}} = \frac{15 \text{ ml}}{20 \text{ mEq}} \rightarrow ? \text{ ml} = \frac{15 \text{ ml}}{20 \text{ mEq}} \times \frac{10 \text{ mEq}}{1} = 7.5 \text{ ml}$$

STRENGTH OF SOLUTIONS-VOLUME/VOLUME

Pure drugs may occur in liquid form. Solid drugs after being diluted become liquid drugs, and, for computation purposes, there is no difference. An example of a liquid drug is Isopropyl Alcohol. A 70% solution of Isopropyl Alcohol can be written as a 70:100 solution. This means that for every 70 parts of pure alcohol there are 100 parts of total solution.

To make a weaker solution from a stronger solution, the nurse needs to remember that "of" means "Multiplied by." For example, "How many ml of 70% alcohol are needed to make 100 ml of a 21% alcohol solution?"

$$? \text{ ml} \times 70\% = 100 \text{ ml} \times 21\%$$

$$? \text{ ml} = \frac{100 \text{ ml} \times 21\%}{70\%} = 30 \text{ ml}$$

For example, "How many ml of a 1:1000 solution are needed to make 20 ml of 1:10000?"

$$? \text{ ml} \times \frac{1}{1000} = 20 \text{ ml} \times \frac{1}{10000}$$

$$? \text{ ml} \times \frac{1}{1000} \times \frac{1000}{1} = 20 \text{ ml} \times \frac{1}{10000} \times \frac{1000}{1} = 2 \text{ ml}$$

Exercise 31

The answers to the following problems are located at the end of this unit. Complete one set of problems, then check your answers. If you are unable to complete the problems *or* if you complete all the sets but don't score 100% on any set, SEE THE INSTRUCTOR. You *do not* need to complete all the sets *if* you can complete a set with 100% correct and understand the principles.

Set 1

(a) A solution contains 50 mg of medication for each 5 ml. How is this concentration described in grams percent?
(b) How many grams of medication need to be added to a diluent to make a liter of 0.3% solution?
(c) You need to add 5 mEq KCl to 500 ml IV fluid. KCl comes in 20 mEq per 15 ml. How many ml should you add?
(d) How many ml of a 50% solution are needed to make 1 L of 10% solution?
(e) How many ml of a 75% solution are needed to make 500 ml of a 25% solution?

Set 2

(a) A solution contains 30 mg of medication for each 2 ml. How is this concentration described in grams percent?
(b) How many grams of medication need to be added to a diluent to make a liter of 30% solution?
(c) You need to add 10 mEq KCl to 500 ml IV fluid. KCl comes in 20 mEq per 15 ml. How many ml should you add?
(d) How many ml of a 40% solution are needed to make 1 L of 20% solution?
(e) How many ml of a 50% solution are needed to make 200 ml of a 25% solution?

Set 3

(a) A solution contains 5 mg of medication for each 1 ml. How is this concentration described in grams percent?
(b) How many grams of medication need to be added to a diluent to make 250 cc of 50% solution?
(c) You need to add 5 mEq KCl to 500 ml IV fluid. KCl comes in 20 mEq per 10 ml. How many ml should you add?
(d) How many ml of a 90% solution are needed to make 1 L of 10% solution?
(e) How many ml of a 75% solution are needed to make 500 ml of a 5% solution?

Answers to Exercises
Exercise 30

Set 1	Set 2	Set 3
(a) 89.6°F = 32.0°C	**(a)** 113.0°F = 45.0°C	**(a)** 96.8°F = 36.0°C
(b) 214°F = 101°C	**(b)** 221°F = 105°C	**(b)** 230°F = 110°C
(c) 38.1°F = 3.4°C	**(c)** 40.3°F = 4.6°C	**(c)** 35.8°F = 2.1°C
(d) 99.2°F = 37.3°C	**(d)** 99.8°F = 37.7°C	**(d)** 92.4°F = 16°C
(e) 58°F = 14°C	**(e)** 70.0°F = 21.1°C	**(e)** 60°F = 16°C
(f) 3.02°F = −16.1°C	**(f)** 4.16°F = −15.47°C	**(f)** 3.28°F = −15.96°C

Exercise 31

Set 1

(a) A solution contains 50 mg of medication for each 5 ml. How is this concentration described in grams percent? 1%

(b) How many grams of medication need to be added to a diluent to make a liter of 0.3% solution? 3 gm

(c) You need to add 5 mEq KCl to 500 ml IV fluid. KCl comes in 20 mEq per 15 ml. How many ml should you add? 3.75 ml

(d) How many ml of a 50% solution are needed to make 1 L of 10% solution? 200 ml

(e) How many ml of a 75% solution are needed to make 500 ml of a 25% solution? 166.67 ml

Set 2

(a) A solution contains 30 mg of medication for each 2 ml. How is this concentration described in grams percent? 1.5%

(b) How many grams of medication need to be added to a diluent to make a liter of 30% solution? 300 gm

(c) You need to add 10 mEq KCl to 500 ml IV fluid. KCl comes in 20 mEq per 15 ml. How many ml should you add? 7.5 ml

(d) How many ml of a 40% solution are needed to make 1 L of 20% solution? 500 ml

(e) How many ml of a 50% solution are needed to make 200 ml of a 25% solution? 100 ml

Set 3

(a) A solution contains 5 mg of medication for each 1 ml. How is this concentration described in grams percent? 0.5%

(b) How many grams of medication need to be added to a diluent to make 250 cc of 50% solution? 125 gm

(c) You need to add 5 mEq KCl to 500 ml IV fluid. KCl comes in 20 mEq per 10 ml. How many ml should you add? 2.5 ml

(d) How many ml of a 90% solution are needed to make 1 L of 10% solution? 111.11 ml

(e) How many ml of a 75% solution are needed to make 500 ml of a 5% solution? 33.33 ml

Work Space

Unit Thirteen
Using Calculators and Computers

Calculators and computers can be a valuable tool in calculating dosages. Today, calculators sell for less than five dollars and are extremely reliable. If the nurse understands some basic facts about calculators, they will make calculating dosages simpler and more accurate.

A basic rule of computing is "GI-GO" (Garbage In-Garbage Out). Unless you put the right information in the computer (or calculator), the answer returned is meaningless. You also have to know what your machine is capable of doing and where there is a strong potential for problems developing.

USING CALCULATORS

Most of today's calculators have five standard keys in addition to the number keys: $+$, $-$, $\div$, $\times$, and $=$. All the calculations used in this book can be done using these fifteen keys. Some calculators have additional keys that may be helpful, but you should not use them unless you are familiar with how they work.

Before starting any calculation, you need to make sure the calculator is starting where you want to begin. Calculators store numbers until they are told to perform a mathematical manipulation with them. If you don't clear the calculator prior to your use, numbers from previous calculations could alter your results. To clear a calculator, either press the clear key twice and then the equal key once or press the equal key twice. The display should then show a 0.

Most calculators only work with decimal fractions. For example, one-half is written as 0.5. This presents problems with fractions like one-third. 0.33333333 is not exactly one-third, so calculations may be slightly off. Most calculators round numbers by stopping when they run out of display space. Try dividing 2 by 3 and you will probably get 0.6666666. Some calculators will round off if the last displayed digit is five or greater. A specific type of calculator, called a *fixed decimal point calculator,* will always give the number to two decimal places. An example of a fixed decimal calculator is a cash register. The answer provided by a cash register is given in cents or hundredths of a dollar. A *floating point calculator* provides a decimal point that moves to the place indicated by the answer.

Calculators normally work on a sequential basis. The numbers are added, subtracted, multiplied, or divided in the order they are entered. One divided by two plus one divided by two is 0.75. Therefore, $\frac{1}{2} + \frac{1}{2} = 1$ must be entered as $1 + 1 \div 2$.

If the number is too large for the calculator to display, an error signal will be displayed and the number displayed can not normally be used. To see your calculator's error signal, fill the display with nines and then multiply by nine. An error signal might also be displayed if an attempt is made to divide by zero.

It is very important to evaluate the answers received from a calculator. Errors frequently made include (1) failing to enter a number or part of a number, (2) using the wrong mathematical process, (3) putting numbers in the calculator in the wrong order, and/or (4) putting the decimal point in the wrong place. Calculators will only help with the implementation stage of mathematical calculations; they will not tell you if you forgot to convert pounds to kilograms. It is usually advised to plan a new calculation on paper first, then use the calculator to add, subtract, multiply, or divide the numbers.

Before you purchase a calculator, know how you are going to use it. If you are going to use it as a staff nurse on evenings and nights, a light-powered calculator will probably not work in the dim lighting. If the calculator is going to go in a uniform pocket, it needs to be small, light, and durable enough to be dropped several times as you search for the narcotic keys. Make sure that the keys can be easily depressed by your fingers and the display is easy to read. If you need a printed record of your calculations, purchase a calculator that uses standard-sized paper and ribbons. A sale calculator today is no bargain tomorrow if you can't find supplies for it.

Test the calculator you plan to purchase by filling the display with a line of 8s. Most displays create numbers by powering a combination of seven straight lines. If all the lines are powered, the figure eight appears. For example:

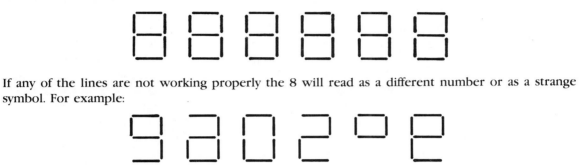

If any of the lines are not working properly the 8 will read as a different number or as a strange symbol. For example:

USING COMPUTERS

Computers are marvelous machines. The material you are reading was written on a computer and proofread by the same machine. Computers are basically giant calculators. When the right number comes up, the printer is told to print a specific letter in a specific place. A *computer program* tells the computer what that number is and what to do when it appears.

The basic usefulness of any computer depends upon the availability of programs. The largest most powerful computer in the world won't do anything without a program telling it what to do. Unfortunately, computers do not speak English. They speak strange languages, and, if they do not understand you, they refuse to cooperate. Most new computer users go through a period of typing in "What do you want?" The computer doesn't answer because it wasn't programmed to reply to "What do you want?" The computer's user needs to know what the computer needs.

Before any computer is purchased, the buyer needs to answer two basic questions: (a) what will the computer be used for and (b) can the task(s) be done cheaper and easier some other way?

What Will the Machine Do?

It is now possible to have a computer terminal at the patient's bedside that records and has access to all the patient's data and also has access to a vast medical and nursing library of information. It is possible to have a program that will prescribe medications, treatments, and tests for a specific patient, taking into consideration all the data from that patient.

While all this is possible, you need to buy a machine based upon the reality, not the possibility. Some computer salespeople will sell you the possibility. It may be possible for a computer to help you learn conversion factors, but the programs aren't written for that specific computer or they are of poor quality. BUY REALITY. If you want a computer to help you learn conversion factors, make sure the programs are available and will work before you buy.

Never purchase a computer based upon equipment or programs that will be available in the future. If a salesperson tells you, "It will be available in two weeks," say, "Wonderful, I'll be back in two weeks." I went back to one store for a year and heard "two weeks" twenty-six times.

Make sure YOU see the machine doing what YOU want it to do while YOU are operating it. You can't take the salesperson to your home or office.

Make sure the machine will continue to perform. Computers sometimes break and computer companies sometimes go out of business. If the tasks you need to do are large enough and/or repetitive enough to require a computer, you don't need a machine that is not repairable or one that must be sent out of town for repairs.

Counting the Cost

Identify all the tasks you want your computer to perform, then ask several salespeople the TOTAL cost of all the equipment, programs, and training necessary to have these tasks done. This is sometimes referred to as a *turn key product*. All you have to do is turn the key and the computer will start performing.

Computer people will want to tell you about RAMs, ROMs, Ks, and all sorts of other computereze terms. It may be helpful to remember that purchasing a computer is like purchasing a car. Few people know what size the piston ring is in the cars they buy. They certainly don't have to know how to change the spark plugs. They do know what they want the car to do in terms of size, status, and comfort. Know what you need to do.

Talk with people who have used computers in order to perform tasks similar to yours. After people have spent a few hundred hours with a particular computer, they learn its strengths and weaknesses. They can also tell you about applications you wouldn't have dreamed of. People who originally purchased computers without disc drives will tell you of the problems of tape storage.

After you have a total price of the system you need—including the computer, monitor, storage device(s), printer, cables, etc.—ask yourself if you could do the job better, faster, and cheaper in some other way. For example, a fairly simple program will convert temperatures from Fahrenheit to Celsius, but, if it only needs to be done occasionally, it can be performed faster and easier with a hand calculator. If you need to calculate all the conversions from $-52°F$ to $200°F$ by $0.2°$ and you have a computer, use it; otherwise, buy a book of conversion factors.

If you can do the tasks you need to do cost effectively with a computer or if your job requires you to use computers, relax. Computers are like combination locks. The first few times they never seem to open even if you think you did everything right. After a while, you can open them without thinking. Just remember two simple rules: (a) back up and (b) evaluate.

"Backing up" is the computereze term for making extra copies of everything. If something can go wrong, it will, and it will generally be when you need the job the most. Backup copies prevent your hard work from being lost to a power surge or careless finger.

Evaluate the results obtained from a computer. Just because a computer performed a drug calculation, doesn't mean you can give 125 g Ampicillin to a newborn. The computer printer probably just skipped the "m" in the milligram abbreviation.

The computer and the calculator are already tools for today's nurse. And they will be as important to tomorrow's nurse as bandage scissors or a stethoscope. But the most important part of good nursing care will always be a logically thinking nurse.

Answers to Pretest Questions
Section I

(1) $\frac{3}{40}$

(2) $\frac{32}{105}$

(3) $\frac{4}{35}$

(4) $\frac{2}{3}$

(5) 4

(6) $\frac{7}{160}$

(7) $\frac{3}{4}$

(8) $\frac{5}{12}$

(9) $1\frac{143}{210}$

(10) $\frac{17}{40}$

(11) $\frac{101}{279}$

(12) $\frac{53}{120}$

(13) $5\frac{50}{99}$

(14) 85.23

(15) 5.2938
(16) 1.7
(17) 42.2422
(18) 18.752
(19) 153.594
(20) 5
(21) 6.2
(22) 0.875
(23) $1\frac{1}{4}$
(24) 60%
(25) 5
(26) 4
(27) $0.50
(28) 7 questions
(29) 18 ounces
(30) 6.25 minutes

Section II

(1) $\frac{1}{2}$ tablets
(2) 2 capsules
(3) 2 tablets
(4) $1\frac{1}{2}$ tablets
(5) 2 capsules

(6) 7.5 ml
(7) 0.7 ml
(8) 10 ml
(9) 4 ml
(10) 1.6 ml

(11) 0.5 ml
(12) 0.8 ml
(13) 1.5 ml
(14) 0.75 ml

Section III

(1) 2 tablets
(2) 0.7 ml
(3) 2 ml
(4) 6 inches
(5) 240 cc

(6) 5 lb 8 oz
(7) 21 gtt/min.
(8) 33 gtt/min.
(9) 125 ml/hr
(10) 1 P.M. or 1300

(11) 25 gtt/min.
(12) 24 gtt/min.
(13) 21 gtt/min.
(14) 25 gtt/min.
(15) 48 gtt/min.

Section IV

(1) 125 mg
(2) 150 mg
(3) 3 ml
(4) 1.5 ml
(5) 10 cc
(6) NO, it is too much.

(7) NO, it is safe.
(8) NO, it is safe.
(9) NO, it is safe.
(10) 75 mg
(11) 1.5 ml
(12) 105.8°F

(13) 89.6°F
(14) 40°C
(15) 30°C
(16) 25 gm
(17) 45 ml

Index